Current Issues in Toxicology

Current Issues in Toxicology

Sponsored by the
International Life Sciences Institute

Edited by H.C. Grice

The Selection of Doses in Chronic
Toxicity/Carcinogenicity Studies

Age-Associated (Geriatric) Pathology:
Its Impact on Long-Term Toxicity Studies

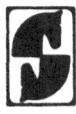

Springer-Verlag
New York Berlin Heidelberg Tokyo

H.C. Grice, *Editor*
Nepean, Ontario, Canada

Library of Congress Cataloging in Publication Data
Main entry under title:
The selection of doses in chronic toxicity/carcino-
  genicity studies ; Age associated (geriatric)
  pathology, its impact on long-term toxicity studies.
  (Current issues in toxicology)
  Includes bibliographies.
  1. Toxicity testing—Addresses, essays, lectures.
2. Poisons—Dose-response relationship—Addresses,
essays, lectures. 3. Carcinogenicity testing—Addresses,
essays, lectures. 4. Carcinogens—Dose-response relationship—Addresses, essays, lectures. 5. Xenobiotics—Metabolism—Age factors—Addresses, essays,
lectures. 6. Rodents—Diseases—Age factors—Addresses,
essays, lectures. I. Age associated (geriatric) pathology, its impact on long-term toxicity studies. 1983.
II. Series. [DNLM: 1. Toxicology. 2. Carcinogens,
Environmental—Administration and dosage. 3. Aging—
Drug effects. QV 600 S464]
RA1199.S44   1983   615.9'07   83-10445

With 3 Figures

9 8 7 6 5 4 3 2 1

ISBN 978-3-540-12845-8   ISBN 978-3-642-49293-8 (eBook)
DOI 10.1007/978-3-642-49293-8

Foreword

The International Life Sciences Institute (ILSI) is a scientific foundation which addresses critical health and safety issues of national and international concern. ILSI promotes international cooperation by providing the mechanism for scientists from government, industry and universities to work together on cooperative programs to generate and disseminate scientific data. The members and trustees of the Institute believe that questions regarding health and safety are best resolved when scientists can examine and discuss issues, as an independent body, separate from the political pressures of individual countries and the economic concerns of individual companies.

Frequently, meaningful assessment of the risk of a test substance is hindered by the inherent inconsistencies in the system. The development and refinement of methods and systems to evelute the safety of chemicals have evolved in a rapid and largely unplanned fashion.

Attempts to improve the system have largely been directed toward broad general concerns, with little attention being given to specific problems or issues. A failure to resolve these problems has frequently resulted in increased testing costs and complications in the assessment and extrapolation of the results.

In response to these difficulties, ILSI has assembled highly qualified and renowned scientists from research institutes, universities, government and industry, with relevant scientific knowledge and expertise regarding the issues that complicate risk assessment procedures.

This series, *Current Issues in Toxicology,* is the result of the endeavors of these international scientists in this regard. It also exemplifies the commitment of ILSI to promote a better understanding of critical safety issues. Throughout this series, an attempt is made to not only examine the factors which influence the evaluation of the safety of chemicals but also to develop principles, recommend guidelines and define areas requiring additional research.

Contents

Current Issues in Toxicology

The Selection of Doses in Chronic Toxicity/Carcinogenicity Studies

Editor in Chief
Dr. H.C. Grice, Scientific Coordinator, International Life Sciences Institute, Nepean, Ontario, Canada

Associate Editors
Dr. D.L. Arnold, Bureau of Chemical Safety, Health and Welfare Canada, Ottawa, Ontario, Canada

Dr. H. Blumenthal, Bureau of Foods, Department of Health and Human Services, Food and Drug Administration, Washington, D.C., U.S.A.

Dr. J.L. Emmerson, Director, Toxicology Studies, Lilly Research Laboratories, Eli Lilly and Company, Greenfield, Indiana, U.S.A.

Dr. D. Krewski, Environmental Health Directorate, Health and Welfare Canada, Ottawa, Ontario, Canada

Contributors

D.L. Arnold, Ph.D.
HPB, Health and Welfare Canada
Ottawa, Canada

R.G. Carlson, D.V.M., Ph.D.
Upjohn International, Inc.
Kalamazoo, Michigan, U.S.A.

Yin Dai, Ph.D.
Chinese Academy of Medical Science
Beijing, China

J.L. Emerson, D.V.M., Ph.D.
The Coca-Cola Company
Atlanta, Georgia, U.S.A.

L. Fishbein, Ph.D.
National Center for
   Toxicology Research
Jefferson, Arkansas, U.S.A.

S. Garattini, M.D.
Instituto di Ricerche Farmacologiche
Milan, Italy

H.C. Grice, D.V.M., M.Sc., V.S.
International Life Sciences Institute
Ottawa, Canada

R. Hess, M.D.
CIBA Geigy AB
Basel, Switzerland

J.C. Kirschman, Ph.D.
General Foods Corporation
Tarrytown, New York, U.S.A.

D. Krewski, Ph.D.
HPB, Health and Welfare Canada
Ottawa, Canada

R. Kroes, D.V.M., Ph.D.
Institute CIVO Toxicology and
   Nutrition TNO
Zeist, Netherlands

I.C. Munro, Ph.D.
HPB, Health and Welfare Canada
Ottawa, Canada

F.W. Oehme, D.V.M., Ph.D.
Kansas State University
Manhattan, Kansas, U.S.A.

D.V. Parke, Ph.D.
University of Surrey
Surrey, England

J.R. Schenken, M.D.
University of Nebraska
Omaha, Nebraska, U.S.A.

J.W. Stanley, Ph.D.
PepsiCo, Inc.
Valhalla, New York, U.S.A.

R.C. Truhaut, D.Sc.
Université René Descarte
Paris, France

Contents

I. Introduction

1. Objectives of Chronic Toxicity Testing

Increasing public demand for greater assurance of safety regarding chemicals found in the human environment has led, in recent years, to a tremendous increase in research and regulatory activity in the field of toxicology. While the ultimate goal is human health, information for use in the safety evaluation of chemicals is derived primarily from various types of bioassay studies using animal models. The objective of long-term tests in rodents is to assess potential chronic toxicity, including carcinogenicity, which would not be evident in tests of shorter duration.

Of paramount importance in the design of any toxicological study is the selection of appropriate exposure levels. Care in the selection of the dosages will maximize the value of the information obtained and greatly facilitate the interpretation of the study results.

In designing a chronic toxicity/carcinogenicity study, it is important to distinguish between a study intended to define the shape and nature of the dose-response curve for the toxicological endpoint of interest and a study in which the primary objective is simply to evaluate the presence or absence of a particular toxicological effect such as carcinogenicity. Because of the limited amount of information provided by the latter type of study (which typically involves the use of only one or two very high dose levels), it is difficult to estimate potential hazards to man at low levels of exposure. The purpose of this monograph, therefore, is to consider strategies to approach the problem of dose selection, with emphasis on the selection of the dose levels to be used in multi-dose, dose-response studies.

2. Review of Existing Guidelines

Existing guidelines for the selection of dosages to be used in chronic toxicity/carcinogenicity studies have been established largely on empirical grounds. These guidelines are often presented in a pragmatic manner without adequate rationale. Practical constraints imposed by the limited availability of adequate testing facilities and the large number of compounds to be tested have frequently resulted in the use of a limited number of relatively high dose levels.

A summary of the published guidelines on dose selection is given in Table I, "Summary of Existing Guidelines for Dose Selection in Chronic Toxicity

Table I. Summary of Existing Guidelines for Dose Selection in Chronic Toxicity or Carcinogenicity Studies

Reference	No. of dose levels	No. of animals	Guidelines		
			High dose	Low dose	Intermediate doses
Barnes & Denz, 1954	3–4 (Chronic food additive)	5–15 per sex	Produces some toxic reaction. On a body weight basis, up to 100 times greater than the estimated daily intake by man.	Per unit of body weight should be the equivalent of 10 times the calculated daily intake of man.	Decided by experimentor.
Fitzhugh, 1955	3	At least 25 (Chronic Study)	Level which approaches the tolerated amount and produces a "menacing" effect on the animals as a whole or on one or more vital organs.	A "no-effect" dosage.	The mid-point between high and low dose.
Clayson, 1962	2 or more (Chem. Carcin.)		The test substance should be presented to the target tissue in as high a concentration as possible without killing or seriously weakening the test animal.		
Della Porta, 1964	2	50 25 are not enough	Should induce some toxic effect, but treatment should be stopped in time to avoid loss of too many animals.		Highest level which will not produce a direct toxic effect.
Abrams et al., 1964	3	50			

Reference	No. of dose levels	No. of animals per group	Criterion	Highest dose level	Dosage relationship / survival
Weisburger and Weisburger, 1967	Minimum 2 (Carcin.)	A statistically adequate number	A certain proportion (10–20%) of the population at risk should succumb to long-term effects.	Should allow extended survival of all the animals.	Relationship between dosages: 1000 (top dose), 500, 100, 50, 10, 5, 1.
Loomis, 1968	6–10	(Chronic) 10	Toxicological signs are necessary, but if toxicity progresses towards lethality, the group is divided into 2 subgroups; one of which no longer receives the test substance.		
	2	(Carcin.) 50 in untreated group; less in treated groups	Evidence of some toxic effect, but as toxic effect becomes evident, administration of test substance is discontinued to avoid loss of too many animals.	The highest dose level which does not produce any direct toxic effects for a period of 50 weeks.	
Berenblum, 1969	Preferably more than 1 (Carcin.)	50–60 or such numbers to yield a significant difference between treated and spontaneous incidence.	The highest that can be tolerated by the animal for long survival when the test substance is administered repeatedly or continuously.		
WHO, 1969	3 (minimum) (Carcin.)	Based on statistical calculation considering (1) spontaneous tumor rate, (2) expected non-tumor death rate,	Should be within the toxic range but should be consistent with the prolonged survival of a majority of the animals.	Should permit the animals to survive in good health for their natural life span or until tumors develop.	Should permit the animals to survive in good health for their natural life span or until tumors develop.

Table I. (*Continued*)

Reference	No. of dose levels	No. of animals	High dose	Low dose	Intermediate doses
		(3) detecting treatment differences.			
Benitz, 1970	(Chronic) (minimum of 3)	20–30 for treated groups; 40–60 for untreated	Should produce definite, harmful effects that serve as an indication of toxicity to be looked for and avoided in man.	Should not produce any adverse physiological, biochemical, or morphological effects and can be used to approximate the margin of safety.	Related to the high and low dose in geometric progression.
Magee, 1970	(Carcin.) 2–3	A statistically meaningful sample size when the animals reach the tumor-bearing age.	As high as can be administered without materially reducing the life span of the animals.	If two dose levels employed, $\frac{1}{4}$ to $\frac{1}{3}$ of maximum; if three dose levels, $\frac{1}{3}$ and $\frac{1}{9}$ of maximum dose.	
FDA Panel, 1971	Several	Depends upon incidence of spontaneous tumors—no hard and fast rule can be laid.	Doses chosen so that they result in experimental conditions likely to yield maximum tumor incidence. Dose which is several orders of magnitude above actual use level.		
D'Aguanno, 1974	3		Expected to produce some toxicity.		
Peck, 1974	2 or 3	25–50 (The larger no. is more appropriate.)	Largest amount tolerated without observable toxic effects, including depressed growth	For drugs, it should be near the therapeutic dose for man.	Midway between high and low.

Guidelines

rate or decreased feed intake, as determined in studies of 3 to 12 months duration (Drug Studies).

Friedman, 1974	At least 3	(a) Will not produce weight depression of more than 10% vs. controls (rodents); nor a weight difference of 10% between control and treated animals of other species. (b) Allows for at least 50% of the treated animals to survive to the end of the study, provided that intercurrent infections do not reduce viability of the test animals. (c) Will not produce pharmacologic effects that will interfere with completion of the study or otherwise invalidate the result.	Must in some way approximate the human use level.	0.10-0.5% high dose.
Health & Welfare Canada, 1975	At least 3	Should not markedly shorten the life span of the animals compared to controls but should be sufficiently high to produce slight but noticeable effects on weight gain, food consumption or some other relevant physiological parameter.	Produces no real increase in tumor incidence over control animals.	

Table I. (*Continued*)

Reference	No. of dose levels	No. of animals	Guidelines		
			High dose	Low dose	Intermediate doses
Newberne, 1975	2 or 3	50	Just under the toxic level.	Some multiple of the dose intended for use in the field or some arbitrary level based on other considerations.	
Sontag *et al.*, 1976	At least 2	50 (Chronic)	Maximum tolerated dose (MTD); should not alter the animals' normal longevity from effects other than carcinogenicity causes; no more than a 10% weight decrement compared to appropriate control group; does not produce mortality, clinical signs of toxicity, or pathologic lesions (other than those that may be related to neoplastic response) that would be predicted to shorten the animals' natural life spans.		0.5 MTD; 0.25 MTD.
Page, 1977a,b	3 (Chronic) (minimum) 1 (Carcin. potential) 2 (Carcin.)		Must be well selected. Maximum tolerated dose.		Fraction of maximum tolerated dose.

	Several— when testing for risk estimation	Maximum tolerated dose; can produce slight toxic effects such as a depression of weight gain.	A minimum of two levels, to span the different toxicological effects observed and to establish useful dose-response information and application of risk-analysis models.
	3 (routine testing for carcinogenicity)	50	
FSC, 1978	4 (minimum) (Chronic)	50 (minimum)	That dose in a subchronic (90 day) study which: (1) induces no overt toxicity, i.e., appreciable death of cells or organ dysfunction as determined by appropriate clinical pathological or biochemical methods; (2) induces no toxic manifestations which are predicted to shorten the life span of the animals except as the result of neoplastic development; (3) in two-generation studies, is not detrimental to conception rates, fetal or neonatal survival, or post-natal development; (4) does not retard weight gain during the subchronic test by greater than 10% as compared to control animals; and	Nonzero response rate.

Table I. (*Continued*)

Reference	No. of dose levels	No. of animals	Guidelines		
			High dose	Low dose	Intermediate doses
			(5) takes into consideration metabolic and pharmacokinetic data, and if dose-dependent qualitative or quantitative differences occur, at least one test dose should be set above the metabolic shift.		
WHO, 1978	Minimum 3 3 (Chronic)	Sufficient numbers to ensure that a statistically valid design is achieved.	Should produce some slight evidence of toxicity, but should be compatible with normal physiological function.	Would not be expected to produce evidence of toxicity.	
Department of Health and Social Security, 1979	Minimum of 3	Minimum of 50 (Chronic)	Just within the toxic range (e.g., a level which causes 10% reduction in body weight gain and/or minimal target organ toxicity).		
	1 or 2	(Carcin.)	Maximum tolerated dose	0.5 MTD or 0.25 MTD	
EPA, 1979	At least 3 (Carcin.)	50 minimum	Induces demonstrated but only slight toxicity and no substantial reduction in longevity due to effects other than tumors.	Less than 0.5 intermediate dose but not less than 0.10 high dose.	0.25 to 0.5 high dose.
	Minimum 3 (Chronic)	58			

| IRLG, 1979 | More than 1 | (Carcin.) Ideally, the number of animals required to provide adequate negative evidence would be such that an excessive risk would not arise if the test failed to detect carcinogenicity. | Estimated maximum tolerated dose—a dose which can be administered for the lifetime of the test animal and not produce:

(1) clinical signs of toxicity or pathologic lesions other than those related to a neoplastic response, but which may interfere with the neoplastic response;

(2) alteration of the normal longevity of the animals from toxic effects other than carcinogenesis; and

(3) more than a relatively small percent inhibition of normal weight gain (not to exceed 10%). |
| CEC, 1980 | 3 | | (Carcin.) One which in subchronic tests induces no overt toxicity or toxic manifestations, and is predicted not to shorten the life span of animals except as a result of neoplastic development. It should not retard weight gain by more than 10% as compared to control.

(Two generation Carcin.) Should not be detrimental to conception rates, fetal or neonatal survival or post-natal development. |

Table I. (*Continued*)

Reference	No. of dose levels	No. of animals	Guidelines		
			High dose	Low dose	Intermediate doses
OECD, 1981	3 (risk assessment)	Each group (dose and concurrent control) should contain at least 50 animals of each sex. (Carcin.)	Elicit some signs of toxicity without causing excessive lethality (chron.-tox.), or without substantially altering the normal life span due to effects other than tumors (carcin.). Signs of toxicity are those that may be indicated by alterations in serum enzyme levels or slight depression of body weight gain (less than 10%). For diet mixture the ingested concentration should not exceed 5%.	Should not interfere with normal growth, development and longevity of the animal; it must not otherwise cause any indication of toxicity. In general, not lower than 0.10 high dose.	Mid-range between high and low doses, depending upon the toxicokinetic properties of the chemical if known.
IARC, 1980	3 minimum (Chronic)	50 minimum	Elicit some toxicity when administered for the duration of the test period, but does not induce: (1) overt toxicity (i.e., appreciable death of cells or organ dysfunction as determined by appropriate methods); (2) toxic manifestations which are predicted materially to reduce the life span of the ani-		Scaled from high dose using factors of 3, 5 or 10.

2 (Carcin.)	mals except as the result of neoplastic development; or (3) 10% or greater retardation of body weight gain as compared with control animals.	0.5 high dose or 0.25 high dose (cancer).
(Two generation)	Should not be significantly detrimental to conception rate, fetal or neonatal survival, or post-natal development. In this respect it may be necessary to use two different dosage schedules: one during reproduction and one during long-term exposure.	

Note: Additional guidelines primarily concerning the conduct of chronic toxicity or carcinogenicity studies include: Bourke, 1955; Shubik and Sice, 1956; Arcos *et al.*, 1968; Boyland, 1968; Shubik, 1970; Roe and Tucker, 1973; Berliner, 1974; Golberg, 1975; Munro, 1977; Rall, 1977; Shubik and Clayson, 1976; Shubik, 1977; Salsburg, 1978; Swenberg, 1979; Fishbein, 1980; Weisburger, 1981.

or Carcinogenicity Studies." A review of these guidelines indicates that the induction of some form of toxicological response is a usual criterion in the selection of the high dose, regardless of the nature of the test substance or whether the study is intended to assess chronic toxicity or carcinogenic potential. Except for carcinogenicity studies involving only one or two doses, it is generally recommended that the lowest test dose should elicit few if any toxicological effects.

3. Overview of the Problems Involved in Dose Selection

Toxicologists have traditionally used doses well in excess of realistic human exposure levels in animal testing for several reasons. Because only a small number of animals can be tested in comparison with the size of the human population potentially exposed to many chemicals, it is considered prudent to use high dosages to ensure that all important toxic effects are elicited. Toxicity testing, by its very nature, involves the application of sufficiently high doses to ensure, beyond reasonable doubt, that the toxic potential of the test substance has been adequately studied and evaluated. The use of high doses will also permit a determination of the nature and degree of adverse effects the chemical is capable of producing.

While adverse effects are usually due to the direct action of the test compound in short-term animal studies of only a few weeks duration, such may not be the case in long-term chronic toxicity/carcinogenicity bioassays. This is because administration of high doses of foreign chemicals or complex mixtures of substances to animals over prolonged periods of time may interfere with normal physiological mechanisms leading to secondary toxic effects. These effects may be induced by a variety of mechanisms, many of which demonstrate apparent thresholds. However, such effects would be invoked only at doses far in excess of human exposure levels (Truhaut, 1980). An example of this phenomena is the production of calculi in the urinary tract of rats by high doses of nitriloacetic acid which leads to the induction of tumors of the kidney (Anderson and Kanerva, 1978). It is also believed that administration of high doses of chemicals that produce chronic liver injury in animals will lead, in some instances, to the induction of liver tumors (Shank and Barrows, 1981). These so-called secondary effects are thought to arise from a variety of causes, including physiological or biochemical alterations in normal organ function, chronic physical injury, prolonged immunosuppression, chronic and excessive hormonal stimulation or nutritional imbalance. The fact that certain chemicals appear to induce tumors through secondary mechanisms has led many toxicologists to criticize the establishment of regulatory standards on the basis of information from such testing programs.

The ability to distinguish between different mechanisms of tumor induction will be enhanced through the inclusion of multiple dose groups spanning a suitable range of doses in the study. While most authorities agree on the need to limit the magnitude of the highest test dose, the criteria for establishing this actual level will vary. It is also clear that the problem is not only one of experimental design, but equally, or more so, one of interpreting the results of high dose testing. A suitable number of dose levels spanning effect and no-effect levels must be employed in order to elicit the spectrum of toxicological effects necessary for the construction of meaningful dose-response relationships which will permit the proper interpretation of the study results.

The remainder of this monograph will focus upon the nature of the information required to select proper doses to be used in long-term studies. Thus, the following questions will be addressed. How many doses should be used? What should the actual dose levels be? What fraction of the available animals should be assigned to each dose? For the most part, this involves a systematic evaluation of all available information on the test substance concerning its use, physical and chemical properties, subchronic toxicity, genotoxicity, and kinetic and pharmacological properties. In addition, consideration will be given to the animal model, duration of test, route of exposure and dosing regimen. Major determinants in selecting the actual levels of exposure include the pharmacokinetic, pharmacological, biochemical, toxicological and nutritional characteristics of the test substance. Consideration will also be given to the selection of dosages for purposes of quantitative risk assessment as well as the doses to be used in special studies such as those involving *in utero* exposure.

It is clear that the selection of doses for use in toxicity studies will require the cooperation of a number of specialists each of whom is responsible for supplying information critical to the selection of the exposure levels to be used and the subsequent interpretation of the study results. While certain guiding principles on the use of this information in selecting an appropriate number and range of dose levels will be presented, it must be recognized that informed scientific judgement must always be applied in order to establish the most suitable protocol to be employed in any particular case. Finally, it is recognized that the procedures for dose selection outlined herein represent an ideal which may not always be achievable in practice.

II. Factors Relating to the Dose Selection

1. Physical and Chemical Properties of the Test Compound

Adequate knowledge of the test chemical's structure, physical and chemical properties, purity and stability is required in dose selection as well as in the development of the study protocol and evaluation of the study results. Unfortunately, this type of information is often not available for test substances present in complex mixtures, the structures of which may never be completely elucidated.

Knowledge of a test chemical's structure may be used for purposes of comparative toxicological evaluation based on the existing toxicological literature pertaining to structural analogs of the test chemical (OTA, 1981). Insight into the relative toxicity of such analogs, as well as some indication as to the nature and site of the toxicological manifestations that could be expected, assists in dose selection and the development of analytical procedures to determine tissue concentrations or metabolites.

Aspects of the chemical and physical property of test substances that could affect the development of the protocol and the interpretation of the experimental results include the following:

Impurities. Impurities or manufacturing by-products at the parts-per-million level often have toxicological effects which could mistakenly be attributed to the test material, such as dioxin in the herbicide 2,4,5-T (FSC, 1978). The purity of commercial food additives and pesticides are often specified by federal or international regulatory agencies. In some instances, the purity of a food additive may be as low as 85% while the active ingredient in many pesticides constitutes an even smaller proportion of the commercial formulation. In the latter situation, the high dose required in the chronic toxicity/carcinogenicity study to produce a toxicological effect may be so great that the effects induced are due to secondary mechanisms or the "non-active" components. Some organizations and agencies have recommended that all toxicological evaluations be conducted using materials that meet the appropriate regulatory requirements for purity (FSC, 1978; WHO, 1967, 1978). Initial toxicological tests should be conducted using the commercial grade of the test material. However, if adverse toxicological effects occur which would preclude or limit its commercial use, then alternative test strategies are required if commercial interest in the test material warrants. An initial alternative might involve the toxicological evaluation of a purer batch of the test material. Subsequently, it may be necessary to conduct studies which provide some degree of assurance to a regulatory agency that the adverse toxicological effects observed in the initial test were solely attributable to removeable impurities.

Reactivity and Stability. Factors related to the reactivity or stability of the test material under conditions of storage or administration (such as chelation, binding with micro- or macromolecules and chemical interactions) can alter the amount of test material received by the animal or produce a new toxic moiety (FSC, 1978). Therefore, appropriate precautions should be taken to ensure that the test animal is indeed being exposed to the test material *per se*, and that the effective dose level is the one intended (Munro, 1977; Burchfield *et al.*, 1977; Page, 1977 a,b; FSC, 1978; Bowman, 1979; IARC Supplement, 1980).

Volatility. While volatility is a desirable property for inhalation studies, the administration of a highly volatile test substance in the diet will dramatically affect the dose level received by the test animal (Jones *et al.*, 1971). If it is appropriate to administer a volatile test material in the diet or drinking water, then precautions must be taken to ensure that the control animals are not exposed via the respiratory route.

Particle size, shape and density. These factors will determine the site of deposition as well as rates and mechanisms of clearance from the respiratory tract (Hatch and Gross, 1964) and absorption in the intestine (WHO, 1978).

Specifications. The chemical specifications and purity of the test compound should be documented. In addition, the stability of the test material *per se,* as well as its stability in the dosing media throughout the period of exposure must be established. Consideration must also be given to compounds that are not discretely identifiable or those in which the material of interest comprises only a small component of the test substance (e.g., amidated pectin, modified starch, irradiated foods).

2. Human Exposure

To the extent possible, the actual dosing regimen and route of exposure employed in the test species should approximate those in man. In general, one of the low doses for any chemical or test substance should be selected so as to produce no anticipated observable toxicological effects. In the case of food additives and pesticides inducing toxicological effects other than cancer, ideally this dose should be sufficiently great so as to permit the application of a suitable safety factor. This is done in order to establish an acceptable level of exposure for man that will not unduly restrict the use of the compound (Vettorazzi, 1980).

3. Acute Toxicity Studies

When toxicological data concerning a test substance are lacking, an acute toxicity study is conducted to assess its relative toxicity and to determine its mode of action on the organ systems affected (Litchfield and Wilcoxon, 1947; Miller and Tainter, 1944; Thompson, 1947; Weil, 1952). The acute study also provides a basis for selecting the doses to be used in short-term toxicity studies.

In recent years, there has been a trend particularly in the drug field to do dose-ranging studies with no attempts being made to provide a definitive LD_{50}. Zbinden and Flury-Roversi (1981) in a detailed review of the significance of the LD_{50}, provide convincing arguments for its replacement with other acute studies that provide more meaningful and useful information.

4. Subchronic Toxicity Studies

Subchronic toxicity studies as discussed here include tests of less than 90 days duration. These are the best guide to dose selection for chronic studies and provide greater insight into the organ systems effected. For chemicals which are rapidly excreted and do not accumulate in body tissues, a study of 2-3 weeks duration should allow the establishment of the dosages to be used in longer studies lasting about 90 days. Effects on reproductive function which are of importance in long-term two-generation bioassays may be ascertained through separate reproductive studies. These longer term studies may involve biochemical and hematological evaluations, the determination of the concentration of the test compound and its metabolites in various tissues or body fluids for a study of the relationship of tissue concentration to the presence of toxicological lesions, interim kills to study the progressive pathogenesis of histological lesions, and the discontinuation of exposure to the test substance in order to assess reversibility.

One consideration in the design and conduct of toxicological studies that is often overlooked, but which has a significant impact upon dose selection in subsequent studies is a comprehensive animal health monitoring program (Arnold et al., 1977; Fox et al., 1979). Such a program can provide an astute investigator with a good understanding of the nature and extent of the clinical toxicity and the varying degrees of toxicity at different dose levels.

One of the objectives of the subchronic study is to establish a "no observed adverse effect level" on the basis of the above observations. Additional observations should permit an accurate determination of the primary target organs affected by the test substance as well as the differentiation between primary effects and those due to secondary mechanisms (e.g., uremia due to chemically induced nephritis).

Several authors have attempted to use the data obtained in acute, short-term and subchronic studies to establish formulae for dose levels to be used in a chronic study (Weil and McCollister, 1963; Weil et al., 1969; McNamara, 1976). However, the experience of the U.S. National Cancer Institute demonstrates that the ability to predict appropriate doses for chronic toxicity tests based on the results of acceptable subchronic studies may be somewhat limited in some cases (Burchfield et al., 1975). This is particularly true for chemicals which accumulate extensively in body tissues such as halogenated hydrocarbons.

5. Metabolism and Pharmacokinetics

The value of information concerning the metabolism of the test substance has long been recognized. However, only within the last few years have metabolic and pharmacokinetic studies become an integral part of toxicological evaluation (FSC, 1978). While practical limitations of space, time, cost and expertise generally dictate the use of species such as the rat, mouse and hamster for chronic toxicity/carcinogenicity studies, pharmacokinetic and metabolic studies suggest that these species are not always appropriate models for man and that the use of gerbils, ferrets, guinea pigs or larger species may be warranted. A desirable objective of such kinetic studies is thus to identify an animal model whose metabolism and disposition to the test substance, as well as the pharmacological effects induced by the chemical, are similar to those observed or anticipated in man. Although many test guidelines recognize the need for such data, it is difficult to obtain the necessary comparative data in the early stages of the safety evaluation process for a new test substance, since metabolic and pharmacokinetic data in man cannot be obtained until reasonable assurances of human safety are available.

Generally, the route of exposure in the test species should correspond to that of man. The mode or route of administration of the chemical (gavage including tablets or capsules, diet including incorporation via microencapsulation, drinking water, dermal or inhalation) as well as its physical characteristics such as solubility and pH will have a profound effect upon the amount absorbed, the nature and degree of metabolism, tissue concentrations and ultimately toxicity. When a test substance is administered orally its bioavailability has to be confirmed. The determination of bioavailability is based on a comparison of the kinetic parameters obtained after oral and intravenous or intraperitoneal administration of the substance. In this regard, the administration of monosodium glutamate (MSG) by gavage resulted in high peak blood levels of MSG which can never be reached by dietary administration, and the hypothalamic lesions observed with gavage administration of MSG are not observed when MSG is added to the diet (Garattini, 1979).

Consequently, the rate and extent of absorption of a test substance should be evaluated under experimental conditions as close as possible to those proposed for the chronic study, using a sufficient number of animals to ascertain the extent of inter-animal variability. This should be done not only after a single administration of the test substance, but also after repeated doses to permit an assessment of changes in the absorption and disposition that may have been induced by the chemical. In the design of chronic studies some consideration must be given to the possibility that the absorption and disposition of the test substance may well change with age. For instance, one-year-old rats cannot metabolize caffeine as well as three-month-old animals (Latini, 1980a). Similarly, in pregnant animals, metabolism, distribution or excretion may be altered because of the physiological changes associated with pregnancy.

The administration of the test substance to an animal may involve a variety of schedules. When chemicals are given every day, the same dose can be spread over most of the day via addition to diet or drinking water, or the dose can be given in a single administration via gavage or injection. Different dosing regimens do not necessarily produce the same peak blood or tissue levels of a given test substance or its metabolites. Hence, the determination of toxic effects is very much dependent on the dosing regimen used (Withey, 1977, 1978). This is particularly so for substances that are readily excreted, like saccharin (Pantarotto *et. al.*, 1981), but does not make nearly as much difference with highly persistent chemicals such as TCDD (Rose, *et. al.*, 1976).

When a high dose level of a test substance exceeds the capacity of the organism to metabolize or excrete it, the kinetics are said to be dose-dependent. In this case an increase in the administered dose level results in a disproportionately greater increase in plasma concentration or the area under the concentration-time curve (AUC). For a given substance, dose-dependent kinetics may be associated with only certain animal species. For instance, rats show dose-dependent kinetics for caffeine at doses between 1 and 10 mg/kg, while such is not the case for mice, rabbits, guinea pigs, monkeys and man (Garattini, 1980). The point at which dose-dependent kinetics occur should be determined, and doses above and below the apparent metabolic break-point should be included in chronic toxicity studies. While this approach is intended to provide some insight into mechanisms of toxicity, it is important to recognize that the dose above the threshold is, by definition, a dose that exceeds the physiological capacity of the animal to handle the chemical. This fact should be taken into account when an assessment of the toxicity of the chemical and extrapolation of the findings to other species are being made.

When a test substance is administered at dose levels resulting in dose-dependent kinetics, biochemical and physiological changes may be induced, which can lead to marked changes in toxicity and tumorigenicity. For man, it is unlikely that such effects would be reached at the level of general use. Examples include the sustained increase in plasma corticosterone induced by high doses of caffeine in rats (Young and Holson, 1978), increased secretion of pituitary hormones when MSG is given at high doses to neonates but not when it is given with the diet (Garattini, 1979), and marked immunosuppression induced by high doses of saccharin added to the diet (Luini *et al.*, 1981).

The lowest dose level to be used in animals should generally not be less than the pharmacokinetically equivalent human exposure level. For example, diazepam remains in the blood for longer periods in man (elimination half-life or $t_{1/2}$ = 20 h) than in rats ($t_{1/2}$<1 h) following a single dose (Garattini *et al.*, 1973). Caffeine, on the other hand, has a shorter half-life in rats than in man at levels lower than 10 mg/kg, whereas the half lives are comparable at levels above 10 mg/kg (Garattini, 1980).

Although it is widely accepted that toxicological effects are generally dose-dependent, a better measure of exposure may be the actual concentration of a substance in the target tissue (Gehring *et al.*, 1978). The wide variability in absorption, metabolism and excretion of chemicals in various animal species, and within individuals of the same species, makes blood or tissue concentrations a more reliable index of target organ exposure (Young and Holson, 1978). Determination of blood or tissue concentrations of the test substance or its metabolites at different times after its administration permits assessment of the exposure of the organism and at the steady-state level enables the calculation of such parameters as volume of distribution, elimination rates, half-life, AUC, and rates of absorption and elimination. These parameters define, in quantitative terms, the fate of the test substance, and are of use in determining the appropriate duration of the subchronic toxicity tests discussed in the previous section. For example, studies with heavy metals or organochlorine compounds which have long residence times *in vivo* might be extended to obtain a better idea of cumulative toxicity. On the other hand, chemicals with a short half-life, might be assessed in a 7-14 day test.

In some instances, the type of metabolites formed from a particular test chemical may vary considerably among different species. For instance, uracil derivatives are major metabolites of caffeine in the rat but occur in much lesser amounts in monkeys and humans (Latini, 1980b).

In some cases, metabolites may be formed but are undetected because of their high chemical reactivity. Such short-lived metabolites as arene oxides and hydroxylamines may covalently bind to macromolecules such as proteins and nucleic acids giving rise to immunosensitization, cytotoxic or carcinogenic effects. Identification of such metabolites or subtle toxicological manifestations may be necessary for the understanding of the mechanisms of the toxic events seen.

6. Pharmacology and Biochemistry

Animal species frequently exhibit differences in tissue sensitivity to chemicals, so that the same concentration of a toxic moiety at the target organ of different species will not necessarily result in a similar response. For example, rodents are unusually sensitive to the teratogenic effects of corticosteroids (Wilson, 1973), the dog mammary tissue is highly sensitive to the carcinogenicity of progestogens (CSM, 1979), and dog and ferret show a unique hemorrhagic response to estrogens (Hall, 1972). Similarly the benzodiazepine oxazepam requires about a six times higher concentration in rat brain than mouse brain for a similar pharmacological response (Garattini, 1973). For this reason, it may be necessary to decrease or increase the dose level to compensate for unusual species sensitivity.

At high dosages, chemicals may increase or decrease their own toxicity by inhibiting or stimulating drug-metabolizing enzymes, or by affecting physiological changes that alter the route of metabolism (Parke, 1978, 1979). For example, chemicals which are slowly metabolized such as phenobarbitone and DDT, increase their own metabolism by enzyme induction; various tricyclic drugs such as imipramine (von Bahr and Orrenius, 1971) inhibit their own metabolism. Thiocarbonyl or thiophosphonyl compounds such as disulfiram and parathion are metabolized by loss of sulphur which results in the destruction of the enzyme system that catalyzes the reaction (Davis and Mende, 1977). Methylenedioxyaryl compounds are metabolized to carbenes which combine with cytochrome P450 to change the route of metabolism thereby decreasing detoxication and increasing activation (Parke, 1978). Where enzyme induction is present, there is an increased dietary requirement for folate which, if not supplied, prevents continuation of the induction with resultant emergence of toxic effects of the chemical itself, together with effects (anemia, teratogenesis) due to folate deficiency (Labadarios et al., 1978). Enzyme induction may also adversely affect the metabolism of endogenous substrates, such as vitamin D, which may result in additional toxicity (osteomalacia, atherosclerosis) (Christiansen et al., 1973).

High dose levels may also affect the metabolic disposition of a material in other ways, as a result of inherent pharmacological activity. The β_2- adrenergic agent, rimiterol, causes splanchnic shutdown at high doses by virtue of residual a-adrenergic activity, and results in impaired gastrointestinal absorption and hepatic metabolism (Griffin et al., 1974). The potential for such biochemical and pharmacological effects at high dose levels should therefore be fully assessed for the chemical under test to ensure that any anomolous toxicity resulting from the use of high dose levels is appreciated, or that lower doses are chosen to avoid these secondary anomalies.

7. Toxicology

In any toxicological investigation it is essential to ensure that the health of the animals is thoroughly assessed prior to and during the course of the investigation. The first step is the acquisition of healthy test animals (Fox et al., 1979). The program includes comprehensive clinical assessment procedures (Fox, 1977) and a health monitoring system (Arnold et al., 1977).

When organs and tissues responsible for detoxification are found to be damaged in subchronic studies, the dose levels for use in the chronic studies should be reduced. The doses selected for the chronic study should not cause toxicity which might have pronounced secondary effects on parameters such as growth rate, immune status or survivability. This, of course, does not preclude the need for a high dose level capable of causing some toxicological effect in the chronic study.

The requirement for the highest dose level to elicit a toxicological response does present a dilemma for test materials which are relatively nontoxic. In such cases, excessively high dosages often must be administered (which may be several orders of magnitude in excess of conceivable human exposure and adequate safety factors) in order to elicit a response; this in turn can induce secondary toxic changes which may not occur in test animals at lower dosages or in man at any conceivable level of exposure. Consequently, if a threshold is to be demonstrated at all, it is necessary to include a number of doses at lower levels. Current guidelines merely indicate that weight loss should not exceed 10%; however, this recommendation has been empirically derived and passed on from one guideline to the next.

In order to define the high dose for use in chronic toxicity studies which is based on valid scientific grounds, attempts should be made to determine the mechanisms involved in toxic events. For example, when a clinical sign such as weight loss is observed, attempts should be made to determine if this was caused by anorexia, palatability, dysphagia or secondary effects due to diarrhea or nutritional imbalances.

Attempts should also be made to assess genotoxic mechanisms by evaluating existing literature to ascertain whether analogs of the test substance are carcinogens; ascertain whether the test substance binds to macromolecules or can nitrosate; and evaluate the results of mutagenicity assays. If careful assessment of such factors suggests that the test substance is likely to be a genotoxic carcinogen, then there is no need for the highest dose to exceed 5% in the diet or an equivalent intake in water. All of the known carcinogens which operate via a genotoxic mechanism appear to have done so at dietary levels of less than 5% (IARC Monographs, 1972, 1980).

8. Nutrition

The test substance may be administered in the basal diet. One diet which is currently popular is the National Institutes of Health (NIH) open-formula diet (Knapka *et al.*, 1974). A test substance added to the diet may produce nutritional imbalance. Subchronic studies may reveal the short-term nutritional consequences of feeding the test substance at high dose levels. Long-term effects will likely only be found during chronic studies.

When fed at extreme dosages even natural food components and natural body constituents can induce toxicity. Ordinary lactose fed at a level of 50% in the diet of dogs caused a watery diarrhea (Beereboom, 1981). The only other remarkable observation in the study was a decrease in urinary sodium output accompanied by gradual elevation in serum calcium, blood urea nitrogren (BUN) and creatinine. After one year, gross evidence of calcium nephropathy was found in the most hypercalcemic of the dogs, an effect almost certainly related to the prolonged diarrhea and not the exposure to lactose *per se*.

Most test substances will not contribute calories to the diet; therefore animals will ingest more diet in an attempt to satisfy their caloric requirement when a substantial portion of nutrient is displaced by test substances. If caloric intake is sufficient to maintain a growth rate similar to that observed in the concurrent control group, there is probably no need for concern. However, if there is an inability to attain sufficient calories for adequate growth, a reduced lifespan or some more subtle physiological aberration could result. In some cases, caloric intake will be equivalent, but weight gain may be less than that of the control group. This difference may involve nutritional deficiencies, extra energy requirements for excretion, or alterations in gastrointestinal functioning due to mild or moderate diarrhea. If such an effect is seen in subchronic studies the cause should be determined before a chronic study is initiated at the same dose levels.

When the test substance provides calories, the proportion of protein to other caloric sources (carbohydrate and fat) will be altered and the relative intake of vitamins and minerals reduced. This situation is particularly evident when the test substance is a lipid; because of a higher caloric density, food and nutrient intake will be reduced beyond that attributable to dilution of nutrients *per se*. If the difference in feed consumption between the control and test groups in a chronic study was substantial, there could be sufficient grounds for invalidating the study in view of the known influence of diet composition on tumor incidence. The early work of Tannenbaum and Silverstone (1957) illustrated the influence of the protein-calorie ratio on the spontaneous incidence of tumors, an effect since confirmed by Ross and Bras (1976) and others. Gellatly (1975) has established that increased dietary fat concentration increases liver tumor incidence in female mice while the data of Carroll and Knox (1975) suggest a similar effect on breast tumors.

The test substance could interfere with nutrient absorption or metabolism. The degree of such interference could be so severe as to preclude long-term tests at other than very low levels of exposure, or be so slight so as to go undetected unless a battery of sensitive biochemical tests were performed. Whenever clinical or laboratory evidence suggestive of altered nutrient metabolism is found, attempts should be made to determine if the effects are likely to be temporary or progressive.

A test substance may decrease feed or water consumption by decreasing palatability, by rendering the food difficult to eat or through some metabolic effect. A reduction of food intake by whatever mechanism introduces an important variable since it is known that dietary restriction results in enhanced survivability and lower tumor incidence in mice (Carroll and Knox, 1975; Tucker, 1979) and rats (Carroll and Knox, 1975). The "normal" ratio of feed to water intake has been reported to be 1:1.9 (NRC, 1972). Conybeare (1980) examined the effect of quality and quantity of diet on survival and tumor incidence in outbred Swiss mice. Dietary restriction was associated with slightly better survival up to 18 months and with a highly significant decrease in the incidence of neoplasms of all types. If the test substance reduces water consumption, feed consumption and weight gain will also be adversely affected.

The cause and nature of any of the preceding effects should be determined and remedial action taken to prevent a variable from compromising the evaluation and interpretation of the chronic toxicity/carcinogenicity study. Possible remedial actions include reducing the dose level, supplementing the diet with a micronutrient where appropriate, or selecting an alternative mode of administration. The possibility of paired feeding might be considered under some circumstances.

A committee of the National Research Council (NRC, 1978) has made the general recommendation that dilution of natural-ingredient diets should not exceed 10%. Certainly the NIH open-formula diet has sufficient nutrients to permit such a dilution without resulting nutritional deficiencies (Knapka et al., 1974). In general, the potential effects of altered diet composition cannot be easily determined and each case must be individually evaluated.

One apparent solution to the problem of diet dilution, and to a great extent, changes in diet composition, is to abandon the natural-ingredient diet in favor of a purified diet so that the test substance can be substituted for a non-essential macroingredient. A committee of the American Institute of Nutrition (AIN, 1977) has recommended a purified diet that purportedly supports normal growth, reproduction and lactation. Though this particular diet has been shown to be equivalent to the NIH open-formula diet during a six-month test period, practical experience with purified diets has been unsatisfactory. The potential advantages of a satisfactory purified diet, however, leave further investigation of the AIN diet a matter of some interest.

9. Statistics

Since direct estimates of risk at very low levels of exposure would require unmanageably large numbers of experimental animals, such estimates are of necessity obtained by downward extrapolation of the dose-response curve observed within the experimental dose range (Crump, 1979). Statistical procedures for quantitative risk assessment involve a mathematical model relating the probability of a response $P(d)$ to the dose d. Due to the statistical problems inherent in determining thresholds (Schneiderman et al., 1979), only non-threshold models will be considered here. While absolute safety may only be guaranteed at zero dose in the absence of a population threshold, a virtually safe dose (VSD) corresponding to some suitably low level of exposure may still be determined (Cornfield, 1977). Particular dose-response models which have been used in estimating VSD's include the probit, logit, Weibull, gamma multi-hit and multi-stage models. The one-hit model arises as a special case of the Weibull, gamma multi-hit and multi-stage models. The biological bases and statistical properties of these models have been recently reviewed by the Food Safety Council (1980), Krewski and Van Ryzin (1981) and Munro and Krewski (1981).

In attempting to obtain estimates of risk which are as precise as possible, the following questions concerning the experimental protocol need to be considered. How many dose levels should be used? What should the actual dose levels be? What fraction of the available animals should be assigned to each dose level? In order to address these questions, consider first the one-hit model and the special case of zero background. The experimental design which minimizes the experimental error of the maximum likelihood estimator of the VSD under this simple one parameter model has been given by Krewski and Kovar (1982). Provided the total number of animals is reasonably large, the optimal design involves assigning all of these animals to that dose level which will induce an expected response rate of 80%. (If this dose exceeds the maximum dose which is to be administered, the optimal dose would be the maximum tolerable dose.) While knowledge of the dose level corresponding to the 80% response rate is required in order for this result to be applied, this one-dose optimal design is highly robust in the sense that the loss in efficiency is minimal if the dose actually employed is at all close to the optimal dose. Thus, only a rough idea of the optimal dose should be sufficient.

The optimal results discussed above are of limited applicability since the one-hit model will not provide a reasonable fit to those data sets for which the dose-response curve exhibits strong upward curvature. The probit, logit, Weibull and gamma multi-hit models will, however, generally provide reasonable fits to such data within the observable range. Since these models all involve two parameters, the optimal experimental designs will involve two nonzero dose levels d_1 and d_2, in addition to a control or zero dose level d_0 = 0 in order to provide for the possibility of background response (Krewski et al., 1983). An example of such a three dose optimal experimental design for the Weibull models is given in Figure 1, "Optimal Experimental Design for Low Dose Extrapolation of Data on Aflatoxin Induced Liver Tumours," under the assumption that the spontaneous and induced responses occur independently (Hoel, 1980). Under the optimal design shown in Figure 1, the majority of the available experimental animals (46%) would be assigned to the low dose d_1, with 18% and 36% of the animals assigned to d_0 and d_2 respectively. In this case, similar results may be obtained under the probit, logit and gamma multi-hit models.

With the dose levels restricted so as to be below some maximum tolerable dose D, the high dose is generally given by $d_2 = D$ with low dose d_1 depending on the degree of curvature in the dose response curve. On the whole, the use of a fixed 1:2:1 allocation among these three doses appears to provide near full efficiency in practice.

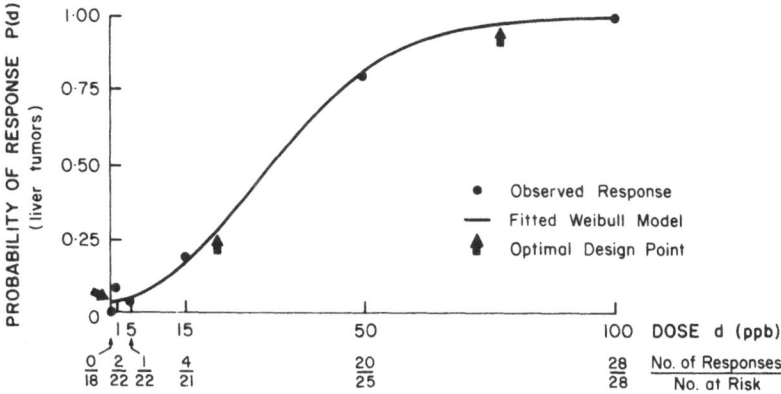

Figure 1. Optimal experimental design for low dose extrapolation of data on aflatoxin induced liver tumors.

An important feature of these designs is that these are also nearly optimal for the linear extrapolation procedure discussed by Van Ryzin (1980). This extrapolation procedure provides for the possibility of low dose linearity and yields conservative estimates of risk at low doses whenever the true dose response curve is actually sublinear in the low dose region.

Since some prior information on the degree of curvature in the dose response curve is required in order to determine the lower of the two positive doses in the three dose designs discussed above, the use of designs involving three or four fixed dose levels and a fixed allocation may also be considered. In practice, a four dose design may actually be preferable in order to protect against the loss of the high dose group due to intercurrent mortality, and allow some assessment of goodness of fit. Among the four dose designs considered by Portier and Hoel (1982) and Krewski *et al.*, (1983), the use of either equally spaced or unequally spaced ($d_0 = 0$, $d_1 = D/4$, $d_2 = D/2$ and $d_3 = D$) doses and either a balanced $1:1:1:1$ allocation or unbalanced $1:2:2:1$ allocation does not appear to be unreasonable for extrapolation purposes.

10. *In Utero* Exposure

Considerable attention is currently being paid by toxicologists to chronic toxicity/carcinogenicity studies involving perinatal exposure of experimental animals to the test substance (Grice *et al.*, 1981). In such studies, the parent or F_0 generation, is dosed with the test substance for some time prior to impregnation as well as during pregnancy and lactation. The offspring or F_1 generation are then dosed with the substance for the remainder of their lifetime or for a substantial period thereof. The second generation is thus exposed to the chemical *in utero* and through the mother's milk (if the chemical gains entrance to the fetus or newborn animal via these routes) as well as through the diet after weaning. Prior to developing a protocol for an *in utero* chronic study, information concerning the subchronic and reproductive toxicity of the compound and its maternal and fetal pharmacokinetic characteristics must be available.

Dose level selection for a two-generation study is particularly demanding since the needs of the dam, neonate, juvenile and F_0 and F_1 adults must be evaluated. Questions which should be addressed include the following: How long prior to breeding should dosing commence? What should the relationship be between dose levels administered to the parent and the offspring in situations where the dam's dose level must be low because of fetotoxic effects? Should the dose level administered to the dam during gestation and lactation be adjusted due to additional caloric requirements? What is an appropriate dose level for a neonate weaned at 21 days of age, when it may have been receiving the test substance from the dam's diet, as well as the unmetabolized or metabolized test substance which may be excreted in the dam's milk? What is an appropriate dose level during the first week or two post-weaning when the animal is rapidly growing and prior to the age when a standard one-generation chronic study would be initiated?

In dealing with new test substances, much of the information needed for dose level selection will be derived from such prechronic studies as the reproduction, teratogenetic and pharmacokinetic studies. These studies will assist in determining dose levels that should be avoided in order to minimize reproductive or teratogenic effects or effects in the F_1 generation that would adversely affect survival. Pharmacokinetic studies will provide information on whether or not metabolic processes in the dam or offspring are saturated. Knowledge of the rate of uptake, the pattern of distribution and the rate of elimination of the test compound is important in determining the effective dose to the conceptus and nursing pups. Pharmacokinetic studies may be used to define the dose level, dosing interval and period of exposure that assures that the dam is in pharmacokinetic equilibrium prior to mating.

In general, the high dose levels administered to the F_0 generation should not markedly affect fertility and the reproductive capability or viability of the offspring. In some instances, the offspring may tolerate a considerably higher dose level than could be administered to the pregnant dams. In such instances the high dose level given to the F_1 might be adjusted upward to comply with generally accepted guidelines on dose selection. However, it should be borne in mind that such a practice may lead to difficulty in assessing and extrapolating dose-response effects, because of the different dose levels administered to the parents and offspring.

III. Principles for Dose Selection

The selection of the most appropriate dose levels to be used in a chronic toxicity/carcinogenicity study is clearly a complex problem. The assembly of the diverse and highly technical inputs that are used in dose selection is time consuming and expensive. Ideally, all of the information discussed in Section II would be obtained in order to establish the most appropriate dose levels. Depending on the objectives of the study, this may not be either feasible or desirable due to time, economic or other constraints. However, it is important that the selection of doses to be used be based on information that will maximize the likelihood that any induced toxic effects are relevant to the safety assessment process, and that the rationale for the dose selection be delineated in the study report to allow for proper evaluation of the study results. The information that will facilitate the selection of the most appropriate dose levels has been detailed in Section II of the monograph. A number of general principles to be followed in dose selection have been derived from a summary of the various sections and are presented below.

Physical and Chemical Properties. Adequate knowledge concerning the chemical and physical properties of the test chemical is necessary for the establishment of appropriate dose levels. Insight into the relative toxicity of analogs of a test chemical as well as some indication as to the nature and site of their toxicological manifestations is helpful in the selection of doses. Knowledge and documentation of the specifications and purity by analysis of the test material are necessary. Establishment of the dosages to be administered to the animals must take into account the fraction of the test material which is represented by the chemical of interest. In addition, the storage stability of the test sample as well as the dosage form throughout the experimental procedure must be established.

Relationship of Doses to Human Exposure. The low dose should be selected so as to produce no toxicological effects in the test animals. This low dose should not be less than the anticipated (pharmacokinetically equivalent) human exposure level and should be sufficiently great so as to permit the application of a suitable safety factor in order to establish an acceptable level of exposure for man. Note that the lowest dose level would be set equal to the human exposure level only when a safety factor of one (1) would be appropriate for the response and chemical under study. To the extent possible, the dosing regimen and route of administration should approximate that in the human situation.

Subchronic Toxicity Studies. Subchronic toxicology studies which define the character of the toxic effects and dose-response relationships are necessary to establish the high doses to be used in chronic toxicity/carcinogenicity studies. The high dose in the chronic study should elicit discernible signs of toxicity but should not alter longevity except due to tumors or unanticipated latent toxic effects.

Metabolism and Pharmacokinetics. Ideally, comparative metabolic and kinetic data should be obtained prior to initiation of the chronic carcinogenicity study. If the dosing regimen and route of administration do not correspond to that in man, the dosing regimen should be adjusted so as to provide exposure levels equivalent to those that would be obtained under the route and regimen applicable in the human situation. If dose-dependent kinetics are evident, then doses both below and above the level at which dose-dependency becomes evident should be employed.

Pharmacology and Biochemistry. Species differences in the sensitivity to the test material may affect the choice of the high dose level. Where the high dose induces changes in the metabolism and disposition of the test substance, the consequences of this must be understood and appreciated.

Toxicology and Pathology. A program conducted by competent personnel to ensure appropriate assessment of the health status of the animals and the diagnosis of disease or toxic states is essential. When effects such as weight loss are observed, attempts should be made to define the etiology in order to assess how such an effect could influence other results of the study.

Nutrition. Nutritional adequacy and fluid balance should be maintained at all dose levels throughout the chronic study. If feed or water consumption are altered, or there is interference with nutrient absorption or utilization, the nature and causes of these effects should be determined. To obtain appropriate safety factors for some macrofeed ingredients, it may be necessary to incorporate them in the diet at levels that exceed 10% of the diet. (Careful consideration should be given when levels over 10% of any substance is added to the basal diet since dilution of essential nutrients is likely.)

Risk Assessment. In the absence of any prior knowledge concerning the shape of the dose-response curve, the use of a control and three test dose levels along with a balanced allocation of test animals may be considered for purposes of quantitative risk assessment.

In Utero Exposure. For *in utero* exposure studies, information from metabolic, reproductive, pharmacokinetic and toxicologic studies is required before informed judgements on dose selection can be made. In general, the high dose administered to the F_0 generation should not markedly alter fertility, reproductive capacity or viability of the offspring. A higher dose may be given to the F_1 offspring although this practice may lead to difficulties in assessing dose-response relationships.

IV. Evaluation and Interpretation of Experimental Findings

Toxicological interpretation and statistical evaluation of experimental results of animal studies rely heavily on the integrity and validity of the available data base. This process is being facilitated through the increasing application of Good Laboratory Practice (GLP) procedures which are now being accepted and practiced on an international scale. In this connection, a critical evaluation of all factors that impinge upon the integrity of the study must be conducted. This will involve an evaluation of the extent to which the protocol was adhered to, how accurately exposure levels were monitored, the general health and survivability of the experimental animals, and the quality of the experimental observations including the histopathological results. The toxicologists, pathologists, statisticians and other scientists who comprise the core team responsible for the design, conduct and evaluation of any study should satisfy themselves, beyond any reasonable doubt, that all the study objectives can be and were achieved.

The process of interpretation involves the assessment of whether or not the substance under test induced any significant toxic effects. These may involve alterations in biochemical or physiological processes including the induction of pathological lesions such as neoplasia. At this stage in the process, it is appropriate to employ statistical procedures to assess the significance of the observed effects as well as evaluate the dose-response characteristics of the test substance and assess the time of onset of any observed toxic effects.

In this connection, judgement must be exercised in determining the biological significance of any induced adverse effects. Once it has been established that a statistically significant and biologically meaningful adverse effect has been induced, it is incumbent upon the investigators to determine, to the extent possible, the mechanism that resulted in the toxic effects in order to determine its relevance to the human situation. In carcinogenicity testing, it is of paramount importance to distinguish when possible between those substances that induce cancer through direct interaction with genetic material and those that induce tumors by overwhelming normal physiological functions.

These questions require a critical evaluation of biological data related to the genetic toxicity, chemical reactivity and other biological characteristics of the test substances. In addition, a careful evaluation of the dose-response characteristics of the test substance is required, including determination of possible threshold effects. This problem of interpretation and extrapolation will be discussed in detail in a subsequent monograph.

V. Recommendations for Future Research on Dose Selection

Dosing Regimen. While most would agree that the route of exposure in the animal should generally correspond to that in the human population, there is no universal agreement as to whether the dose should be on a mg/kg/body weight per day or as a percentage of the diet. The former requires weekly or biweekly adjustments of the diet if the dose level is to be kept constant. Since the actual dose received can vary markedly under these two regimens, particularly for young animals, research as to the most appropriate regimen would be helpful.

Nonlinear Kinetics. Studies should be initiated in order to evaluate the utility of using doses within the region of dose-dependent kinetics.

Quantitative Risk Assessment. Optimal experimental designs for extrapolation procedures utilizing time-to-response information should be considered in addition to those discussed here for quantal response data.

In Utero Chronic Toxicity/Carcinogenicity Studies. In utero, chronic toxicity/carcinogenicity studies provide an additional experimental model for toxicological testing, which may be more appropriate when humans might be exposed *in utero* or for significant segments of their lives. However, further comparative data are required to evaluate fully the appropriateness and the need for such studies in present safety evaluation programs. There is a need to establish guidelines on dose selection for use in *in utero* studies. This should include a consideration of the dose to the dam prior to pregnancy, and during pregnancy and lactation, to the neonate, to the juvenile, and to the adult animal.

Geriatric Animals. There is a need to determine if doses selected on the basis of the pharmacokinetic capabilities of a young healthy animal, are appropriate for a geriatric animal. Several factors have resulted in an increased longevity of animals used in toxicity studies. Suppliers provide healthier animals that are resistant to some of the common diseases of laboratory animals. Improved facilities and animal care have greatly reduced the incidence of intercurrent infections. This increased longevity in laboratory animals is paralleled by an increasing longevity in a greater segment of the human population. It seems reasonable therefore to suggest that animal studies should be of sufficient duration to permit assessment of test chemicals in the geriatric group. However, there is very little information on the changing metabolic capabilities involved in the normal aging process or how diseases of the aged might alter metabolism. How these altered metabolic or disease processes might influence toxicity is largely unknown (Salsburg, 1978).

VI. Summary

This monograph provides some historical background and an overview of the problems involved in dose selection in chronic toxicity/carcinogenicity studies. Consideration is given primarily to the design and protocol aspects of chronic studies relating to dose selection, with some consideration as how these may relate to the interpretation of study results. Existing practices in dose selection have been empirically derived over a number of years. Traditionally, a range of doses has been employed to define levels for which effects are and are not observed. In recent years, very high doses have often been used in an attempt to evaluate the full toxic potential of the test chemical. However, the use of very high doses has come into question with the growing realization that administration of high doses of foreign chemicals to animals over prolonged periods may alter normal physiological mechanisms thereby leading to secondary toxic effects that would not be observed at levels of the chemicals to which humans would be realistically exposed.

The process of dose selection involves the undertaking of preliminary studies by a number of specialists working in concert to provide the information required for the selection of the most appropriate doses. This includes a consideration of the physical and chemical properties of the test chemical, knowledge of purity and impurities, reactivity, and stability under conditions of storage or administration. Factors such as the vapor pressure of a test substance and a knowledge of particle size, shape and density are also important. Preliminary toxicity studies that are required for appropriate selection of doses include acute, short-term and subchronic toxicity and genotoxicity. The studies are usually carried out sequentially and provide information on the nature and extent of the toxic events and the degree of toxicity at different dosage levels. The final selection of high doses for the chronic study needs to take cognizance of such effects and the fact that larger numbers of animals will be on test for longer periods of time.

A number of dose levels spanning the anticipated range of toxicological, pharmacokinetic, pharmacological and biochemical effects should be employed to elucidate the nature of any dose-dependent effects, the shape of the dose-response curve and possible mechanisms of action. The use of a control group and either three or four dose levels is appropriate. The high dose should not adversely affect the nutritional status of the test animals nor alter longevity except due to the induction of tumors or unanticipated latent toxic effects, including immune response. The high dose should not exceed that dose at which toxic effects are noted in subchronic studies and yet it should elicit, if possible, discernable signs of toxicity. The low dose should not be lower than the pharmacokinetically equivalent human exposure level and should, ideally, produce no toxicological effects. Intermediate doses should be selected so as to provide sufficient data for purposes of quantitative risk assessment or the application of suitable factors where appropriate.

VII. Glossary of Terms - As They Pertain to Toxicology

AUC - area under the blood concentration-time curve following the administration of a single oral or i.v. dose of the test chemical. This affords a measure of the total exposure to the test chemical.

Acute Toxicity - studies usually involving a single administration of a chemical and observation of the animal for toxic effects for periods from 7 to 21 days.

Median Lethal Dose (LD_{50}) - that dose which can be expected to produce 50% mortality following acute exposure.

Carcinogenicity Study - is used to indicate a comprehensive multidose long-term study. There is increasing recognition of the need to include adequate dose levels in carcinogenicity studies to permit proper statistical evaluation to include quantitative risk assessment. Because long-term studies are so very expensive to conduct, it is prudent to design studies to meet the requirements for both toxicity and carcinogenicity testing. The preferred term to describe such studies would be a chronic toxicity/carcinogenicity study.

Chronic Toxicity - traditionally these are tests lasting about 24 months in duration. Carcinogenicity is one of the toxic parameters that is taken into consideration.

Genotoxic - effects that adversely alter the genetic material of the cell.

Metabolic Break-Point - for simplicity it is assumed that there are two rate processes involved in the metabolism of a specific substrate, and at low concentration, rate process one predominates by a ratio of 1000:1 over rate process two. When the concentration of the substrate increased to the extent that rate process one is saturated and rate process two increases to the point that the ratio is less than 1000:1, the metabolic break-point has been reached.

Metabolism - the sum of all the physical and chemical processes by which living organized substance is produced and maintained.

Pharmacokinetics - the quantitative and qualitative description of the time course of absorption, distribution, and elimination of an agent in an intact animal.

Quantitative Risk Assessment - the use of mathematical modelling procedures to estimate risks at low levels of exposure outside range actually tested.

Dose-dependent kinetics - a disproportional increase of the half-life or an increase in the area under the curve higher than expected when the dose is increased. This usually involves the kinetics of a test chemical changing from first-order to zero-order rate constants as capacity-limited routes are measured and pathways or systems become saturated by a large dose.

VIII. References

Abrams, W.B., Bagdon, R.E., and Zbinden, G. (1964). Techniques of animal and clinical toxicology. In *Animal and Clinical Pharmacologic Techniques in Drug Evaluation* (J.H. Nodine and P.E. Siegler, eds.) Year Book Medical Publishing Inc., Chicago.

A.I.N. (1977). Report of the American Institute of Nutrition ad hoc committee on standards for nutritional studies. *J. Nutr.* 107, 1340.

Anderson, R.L. and Kanerva, R.L. (1978). Hypercalcinuria and crystalluria during ingestion of dietary nitrilotriacetate. *Food Cosmet. Toxicol.* 16, 569-574.

Arcos, J.C., Argus, M.F., and Wolf, G. (1968). *Chemical Induction of Cancer: Structural Basis and Biological Mechanisms.* Volume I, pp. 340-463, Academic Press, New York.

Arnold, D.L., Charbonneau, S.M., Zawidzka, Z.Z., and Grice, H.C. (1977). Monitoring animal health during chronic toxicity studies. *J. Environ. Pathol. Toxicol.* 1, 227-239.

Barnes, J.M. and Denz, F.A. (1954). Experimental methods used in determining chronic toxicity; a critical review. *Pharmacol. Rev.* 6, 191-242.

Beereboom, J. (1981). Bulking agents and fillers. In *Impact of Toxicology on Food Processing* (J. Ayers and J. Kirschman, eds.) pp. 273-285, AVI Publishing Co. Inc., Westport.

Benitz, K.F. (1970). Measurements of chronic toxicity. In *Methods in Toxicology* (G.E. Paget, ed.) pp. 82-131, Blackwell Scientific Publications, Oxford and Edinburgh.

Berenblum, I. (ed.) (1969). Carcinogenicity testing: a report of the panel on carcinogenicity of the Cancer Research Commission of the UICC. *UICC Technical Report Series,* Vol. 2.

Berliner, V.R. (1974). U.S. Food and Drug Administration requirements for toxicity testing of contraceptive products. *Endocrin.* 75, 240-265.

Bourke, A.R. (1955). VII Carcinogenicity. *Food, Drug, Cosmet. Law J.* 719-721.

Boyland, B. (1968). Carcinogenicity. In *Modern Trends in Toxicology.* Volume I (B. Boyland and R. Goulding, eds.) pp. 107-129, Butterworth and Company, Ltd., London.

Bowman, M.C. (1979). *Carcinogens and Related Substances: Analytical Chemistry for Toxicological Research.* pp. 23-58, M. Dekker, New York.

Burchfield, H.P., Storrs, E.E., and Green, E.E. (1977). Role of analytical chemistry in carcinogenesis studies. In *Advances in Modern Toxicology,* Vol. 3, *Environmental Cancer* (H.F. Kraybill and M.A. Mehlman, eds.) pp. 137-207, Hemisphere, Washington.

Burchfield, H.P., Storrs, E.E., and Kraybill, H.F. (1975). The maximum tolerated dose in pesticide carcinogenicity studies. In *Environmental Quality and Safety, Supplement Vol. III* (F. Coulston and F. Korte, eds.) pp. 599-603, Georg Thieme Publishers, Stuttgart.

Carroll, K.K. and Knox, H.T. (1975). Dietary fat in relation to tumorigenesis. *Prog. Biochem. Pharmacol.* 10, 308-353.

CEC: Commission of the European Communities (1980). Food-science and techniques. Reports of the scientific committee for food (tenth series). *Guidelines for the Safety Assessment of Food Additives.*

Christiansen, C., Modbro, P., and Lund, M. (1973). Incidence of anti convulsant osteomalacia and effect of vitamin D: controlled therapeutic trial. *Br. Med. J.* 4, 695-701.

Clayson, D.B. (1962). Testing chemicals for carcinogenic activity. I. Methods. In *Chemical Carcinogenesis* pp. 55-85, J. and A. Churchill, Ltd., London.

Conybeare, G. (1980). Effect of quality and quantity of diet on survival and tumor incidence in outbred Swiss mice. *Food Cosmet. Toxicol.* 18, 65-75.

Cornfield, J. (1977). Carcinogenic risk assessment. *Science* 198, 693-699.

Crump, K.S. (1979). Dose response problems in carcinogenesis. *Biometrics* 35, 157-167.

CSM: Committee of Safety for Medicines (1979). *Medicine Act Information Letter,* United Kingdom, No. 25, p. 2.

D'Aguanno, W. (1974). Drug safety evaluation - pre-clinical considerations. In *Neuroleptics* (S. Fielding and H. Lal, eds.) pp. 317-332, Futura Publishing Company, New York.

Davis, J.E. and Mende, T.J. (1977). A study of the binding of sulphur to rat liver microsomes which occurs concurrently with the metabolism of parathion. *J. Pharmacol. Exp. Ther.* 201, 490-497.

Della Porta, G. (1964). The study of chemical substances for possible carcinogenic actions. *Proc. Eur. Soc. Study Drug Toxic.* 3, 29-40.

Department of Health and Social Security (1979). Committee on carcinogenicity of chemicals in food: consumer products and the environment. *A Consultative Document on Guidelines for the Testing of Chemicals for Carcinogenicity.* London, as of April, 1979.

FDA: Food and Drug Administration (1971). Advisory committee on protocols for safety evaluation: panel on carcinogenesis report on cancer testing in the safety evaluation of food additives and pesticides. *Toxicol. Appl. Pharmacol.* 20, 419-438.

Fishbein, L. (1980). New concepts of design and utility of large-scale carcinogenicity studies. *J. Toxicol. Environ. Health* 6, 1081-1100.

Fitzhugh, O. G. (1955). VI Chronic oral toxicity. *Food Drug Cosmet. Law J.,* 712-719.

Food Safety Council (1978). Proposed system for food safety assessment. *Food Cosmet. Toxicol.* 16, Suppl. 2.

Food Safety Council (1980). *Proposed System for Food Safety Assessment.* Food Safety Council, Washington.

Fox, J.G. (1977). Clinical assessment of laboratory rodents on long-term bioassay studies. *J. Environ. Pathol. Toxicol.* 1, 199-226.

Fox, J.G., Thibert, T., Arnold, D.L., Krewski, D.R., and Grice, H.C. (1979) Toxicology studies. II. The laboratory animal. *Food Cosmet. Toxicol.* 17, 661-675.

Friedman, L. (1974). Section 4. Report of Discussion Group No. 3. Dose selection and administration. In *Carcinogenesis Testing of Chemicals* (L. Golberg, ed.) pp. 21-22, CRC Press, Inc., Cleveland.

Garattini, S. (1979). Evaluation of the neurotoxic effects of glutamic acid. In *Nutrition and the Brain,* Volume IV (R.J. Wurtman and J.J. Wurtman, eds.) pp. 79-124, Raven Press, New York.

Garattini, S. (1980). Data presented at the International Life Sciences Institute, Third International Caffeine Workshop, Hunt Valley, Maryland, October 27-29.

Garattini, S., Mussini, E., Marcucci, F., and Guaitani, A. (1973). Metabolic studies on benzodiazepines in various animal species. In *The Benzodiazepines* (S. Garattini, E. Mussini and L.O. Randall, eds.) pp. 75-97, Raven Press, New York.

Gehring, P.J., Watanabe, P.G. and Park, C. (1978). Use of dose-response toxicity data for chemicals requiring metabolic acitivation. Example...vinyl chloride. *Toxicol. Appl. Pharmacol.* 44, 581-591.

Gellatly, J.G. (1975). The natural history of hepatic parenchymal nodule formation in a colony of C57BL mice with reference to the effect of diet. In *Hepatic Neoplasia* (W.H. Butler and P.M. Newberne, eds.) pp. 77-109, Elsevier Scientific, Amsterdam.

Golberg, L. (1975). Safety evaluation concepts. Symposium on safety evaluation and toxicological tests and procedures. *J. Assoc. Off. Anal. Chem.* 58, 635-644.

Grice, H.C., Munro, I.C., Krewski, D.R. and Blumenthal, H. (1981). *In Utero* exposure in chronic toxicity carcinogenicity studies. *Food Cosmet. Toxicol.* 19, 373-379.

Griffin, J.P., Williams, J.R.B., and Maughan, E. (1974). The metabolism of rimiterol hydrobromide at different intravenous dose levels in the rat. *Xenobiotica* 4, 755-764.

Hall, D.E. (1972). *Blood Coagulation and its Disorders in the Dog,* pp. 97-101,Bailliere Tindall, London.

Hatch, T.F. and Gross, P. (1964). *Pulmonary Deposition of Inhaled Aerosols.* Academic Press, New York.

Health and Welfare Canada (1975). *The Testing of Chemicals for Carcinogenicity, Mutagenicity, and Teratogenicity.* pp. 2-31, Health and Welfare Canada, Ottawa.

Hoel, D.G. (1980). Incorporation of background response in dose-response models. *Fed. Proc.* 39, 73-75.

IARC: International Agency for Research on Cancer (1980). *Long-term and Short-term Screening Assays for Carcinogenesis: A Critical Appraisal.* Supplement 2, IARC, Lyon.

IARC (1972-1980). *Monographs on the Evaluation of Carcinogenic Risk of Chemicals to Man.* IARC, Lyon.

IRLG: Interagency Regulatory Liaison Group (1979). Work Group on Risk Assessment. Scientific bases for identification of potential. *J. Nat. Cancer Inst.* 63, 241-268.

Jones, W.I., Roback, L.A., and Taylor, J.M. (1971). The loss of food flavours from laboratory animal diets. II. Effect of laboratory environment. *J. Assoc. Off. Anal. Chem.* 54, 42-46.

Knapka, J.J., Smith, K.P., and Judge, F.J. (1974). Effect of open and closed formula rations on the performance of three strains of laboratory mice. *Lab. Anim. Sci.* 24, 480-487.

Krewski, D. and Van Ryzin, J. (1981). Dose-response models for quantal response toxicity data. In *Statistics and Related Topics* (M. Csorgo, D. Dawson, J.N.K. Rao and E. Saleh, eds.) pp. 201-231, Elsevier/North-Holland, Amsterdam.

Krewski, D. and Kovar, J. (1982). Low dose extrapolation under single parameter dose-response models. *Communications in Statistics* Series B, Volume 11. pp. 27-46.

Krewski, D., Kovar, J., and Bickis, M. (1983). Optimal experimental designs for low dose extrapolation. In *Topics in Applied Statistics* (T.W. Dwizedi, ed.)M. Dekker, New York. (in press)

Labadarios, D., Dickerson, J.W.T., Lucas, E.G., Obuwa, G.H., and Parke, D.V. (1978). The effects of chronic drug administration on hepatic enzyme induction and folate metabolism. *Brit. J. Clin. Pharmacol.* 5, 167-173.

Latini, R., Bonati, M., Marzi, E., Tacconi, M.T., Sadurska, B., and Bizzi, A. (1980a). Caffeine disposition and effects in young and one-year-old rats. *J. Pharm. Pharmacol.* 32, 596-599.

Latini, R., Bonati, M., Marzi, E., and Garattini, S. (1980b). Urinary excretion of an uracilic metabolite from caffeine by rat, monkey, man. *Toxicol. Lett.* 7, 267-272.

Litchfield, J.T. and Wilcoxon, F.A. (1947). A simplified method of evaluating dose-effect experiments. J. *Pharmacol. Exp. Ther.* 95, 99-113.

Loomis, T.A. (1968). *Essentials of Toxicology.* pp. 139-156, Lea and Febiger, Philadelphia.

Luini, W., Mantovani, A., and Garattini, S. (1981). Effects of saccharin on primary humoral antibody production in rats. *Toxicol. Lett.* 80, 1-6.

Magee, P.N. (1970). Tests for carcinogenic potential. In *Methods in Toxicology* (G.E. Paget, ed.) pp. 158-196, Blackwell Scientific Publications, Oxford and Edinburgh.

McNamara, B.P. (1976). Concepts in health evaluation of commercial and industrial chemicals. In *Advances in Modern Toxicology, Vol. I. New Concepts in Safety Evaluation* (M.A. Mehlman, R.E. Shapiro and H. Blumenthal, eds.) pp. 61-140, Hemisphere, Washington.

Miller, L.C. and Tainter, M.C. (1944). Estimation of the ED_{50} and its error by means of log-probit graph paper. *Proc. Soc. Exp. Biol. Med.* 57, 261-264.

Munro, I.C. (1977). Considerations in chronic toxicity testing: the chemical, the dose, the design. *J. Environ. Pathol. Toxicol.* 1, 183-197.

Munro, I.C. and Krewski, D.R. (1981). Risk assessment and regulatory decision making. *Food Cosmet. Toxicol.* 19, 549-560.

Newberne, P.M. (1975). Pathology: studies of chronic toxicity and carcinogenicity. *J. Assoc. Off. Anal. Chem.* 58, 650-656.

NRC: National Research Council (1972). *Nutrient Requirements of Laboratory Animals,* No. 10 (2nd revised ed.) National Academy of Sciences, Washington.

NRC: National Research Council (1978). *Control of Diets in Laboratory Animal Experimentation.* National Academy of Sciences, Washington.

OECD: Organization of Economic and Cooperative Development (1981). OECD Long-term Expert Group: *Test Guidelines for Carcinogenicity Studies.*

OTA: Office of Technology Assessment (1981). *Assessment of Technologies for Determining Cancer Risks from the Environment.* U.S. Government Printing Office, Washington.

Page, N.P. (1977a). Chronic toxicity and carcinogenicity guidelines. *J. Environ. Pathol. Toxicol.* 1, 161-182.

Page, N.P. (1977b). Concepts of a bioassay program in environmental carcinogenesis. In *Advances in Modern Toxicology, Vol. 3. Environmental Cancer* (H.F. Kraybill and M.A. Mehlman, eds.) pp. 108-113, Hemisphere, Washington.

Pantarotto, C., Salmona, M., and Garattini, S. (1981). Plasma kinetics and urinary elimination of saccharin in man. *Toxicol. Lett.* 9, 367-371.

Parke, D.V. (1978). The responsiveness of cells to various drug inducers. In *The Induction of Drug Metabolism: Symposium Ashford Castle, Ireland* (R.W. Estabrook and E. Lindenlaub, eds.) pp. 133-150, Schattauer Verlag, Stuttgart.

Parke, D.V. (1979). Toxicological consequences of enzyme induction and inhibition. In *Aspects of Drug Toxicity* (J.W. Gorrod, ed.) pp. 101-111, Taylor and Francis, London.

Peck, H.M. (1974). Design of experiments to detect carcinogenic effects of drugs. In *Carcinogenesis Testing of Chemicals* (L. Golberg, ed.) pp. 1-13, CRC Press, Inc., Cleveland.

Portier, C. and Hoel, D. (1982). Technical report on bioassay design. *Technical report,* National Institute of Environmental Health Services, Research Triangle Park.

Rall, D.P. (1977). Species differences in carcinogenesis testing. In *Origins of Human Cancer* (H.H. Hiatt, J.D. Watson, and J.A. Winsten, eds.) pp. 1383-1390, Cold Spring Harbor Laboratory, New York.

Roe, F.J.C. and Tucker, M.J. (1973). Recent developments in the design of carcinogenicity tests of laboratory animals. *Proc. Eur. Soc. Study Drug Toxic.* 15, 171-177.

Rose, J.Q., Ramsey, J.C., Wentzler, T.H., Hummel, R.A., and Gehring, P.J. (1976). The fate of 2,3,7,8-tetrachlorodibenzo-p-dioxin following single and repeated oral doses to the rat. *Toxicol. Appl. Pharmacol.* 36, 209-226.

Ross, M.H. and Bras, G. (1976). Influence of protein under - and over - nutrition on spontaneous tumor prevalence in the rat. *J. Nutr.* 250, 263-265.

Salsburg, D. (1978). Lifetime carcinogenic studies in rodents, viewed from the standpoint of experimental design: weaknesses and alternatives. In *Carcinogenicity Testing: Principles and Problems* (A.D. Dayan and R.W. Brimblecombe, eds.) University Park Press, Baltimore.

Schneiderman, M.A., Decoufle, P., and Brown, C.C. (1979). Thresholds for environmental cancer: biologic and statistical considerations. *Ann. N.Y. Acad. Sci.* 329, 92-130.

Shank, R.C. and Barrows, L.R. (1981). Toxicity-dependent DNA methylation: significance to risk assessment. In *Health Risk Analysis* (C.R. Richmond, P.J. Walsh and E.D. Copenhaver, eds.) pp. 225-233, Franklin Institute Press, Philadelphia.

Shubik, P. (1970). Symposium on the evaluation of the safety of food additives and chemical residues: III. The role of the chronic study in the laboratory animal for evaluation of safety. *Toxicol. Appl. Pharmacol.* 16, 507-512.

Shubik, P. (1977). General criteria for assessing the evidence for carcinogenicity of chemical substances: report of the Subcommittee on Environmental Carcinogenesis, National Cancer Advisory Board. *J. Nat. Cancer Inst.* 58, 461-465.

Shubik, P. and Clayson, D.B. (1976). Application of the results of carcinogen bioassays to man. In *Environmental Pollution and Carcinogenic Risks,* International Agency for Research on Cancer. Scientific Publications No. 13, Lyon.

Shubik, P. and Sice, J. (1956). Chemical carcinogenesis as a chronic toxicity test. *Cancer Res.* 16, 728-742.

Sontag, J.M., Page, N.P., and Saffioti, U. (1976). *Guidelines for Carcinogen Bioassay in Small Rodents.* DHEW Publication No. 76-801.

Swenberg, J.A. (1979). Incorporation of transplacental exposure into routine carcinogenicity bioassays. *Nat. Cancer Inst. Monogr.* 51, 265-268.

Tannenbaum, A. and Silverstone, H. (1957). Nutrition and genesis of tumors. In *Cancer,* Volume I (R.W. Raven, ed.) pp. 306, Butterworth and Co. Ltd., London.

Thompson, W. (1947). Use of moving averages and interpolation to estimate median effective dose. *Bac. Rev.* 11, 115-141.

Truhaut, R. (1980). The problem of thresholds for chemical carcinogens - its importance in industrial hygiene, especially in the field of permissible limits for occupational exposure. *Am. Ind. Hyg. Assoc. J.* 41, 685-692.

Tucker, M.J. (1979). The effect of long term food restriction on tumours in rodents. *Int. J. Cancer* 23, 803.

Van Ryzin, J. (1980). Quantitative risk assessment. *J. Occup. Med.* 22, 321-326.

Vettorazzi, G. (1980). *Handbook of International Food Regulatory Toxicology. Vol. I. Evaluations.* Spectrum Publication, Jamaica, New York.

von Bahr, C. and Orrenius, S. (1971). Spectral studies on the interaction of imipramine and some of its oxidized metabolites with rat liver microsomes. *Xenobiotica* 1, 69-78.

Weil, C.S. (1952). Tables for convenient calculation of median effective dose (LD_{50} or ED_{50}) and constructions in their use. *Biometrics* 8, 249-263.

Weil, C.S. and McCollister, D.D. (1963). Relationship between short and long-term feeding studies in designing an effective toxicity test. *Agric. Food Chem.* 11, 486-491.

Weil, C.S., Woodside, M.D., Bernard, J.R., and Carpenter, C.P. (1969). Relationship between single-peroral, one-week and ninety-day rat feeding studies. *Toxicol. Appl. Pharmacol.* 14, 426-431.

Weisburger, E. (1981). Techniques for carcinogenicity studies. *Cancer Res.* 41, 3690-3694.

Weisburger, J.H. and Weisburger, E.K. (1967). Tests for chemical carcinogenesis. In *Methods in Cancer Research* (H. Busch, ed.) Vol. 1, pp. 307-398, Academic Press, New York.

WHO (1967). Procedures for investigating intentional and unintentional food additives. Report of a WHO scientific group. *World Health Organization Technical Report Series, No. 348.* Geneva.

WHO (1969). Principles for the testing and evaluation of drugs for carcinogenicity. Report of a WHO scientific group. *World Health Organization Technical Report Series, No. 426.* Geneva.

WHO (1978). Principles and methods for evaluating toxicity of chemicals, Part 1. *Environmental Health Criteria, Vol. 6,* World Health Organization, Geneva.

Wilson, J.G. (1973). Present status of drugs as teratogens in man. *Teratology* 7, 3.

Withey, J.R. (1977). The role of pharmacokinetics in the design and conduct of chronic exposure studies. *Excerpta Med. Int. Cong. Ser.,* No. 440, 190-195.

Withey, J.R. (1978). Pharmacokinetic principles. In *Proceedings First International Congress on Toxicology: Toxicology as a Predictive Science* (G.L. Plaa and W.A.M. Duncan, eds.) pp. 119-141, Academic Press, New York.

Young, J.F. and Holson, J.F. (1978). Utility of pharmacokinetics in designing toxicological protocols and improving interspecies extrapolation. *J. Environ. Pathol. Toxicol.* 2, 169-186.

Zbinden, G. and Flury-Roversi, M. (1981). Significance of the LD_{50}-test for the toxicological evaluation of chemical substances. *Arch. Toxicol.* 47, 77-99.

Age-Associated (Geriatric) Pathology:
Its Impact on Long-Term Toxicity Studies

Editor in Chief
Dr. H.C. Grice, Scientific Coordinator, International Life Sciences Institute, Nepean, Ontario, Canada

Associate Editor
Dr. J.D. Burek, Senior Director of Safety Assessment, Merck Sharp and Dohme Research Labs, West Point, Pennsylvania, U.S.A.

Contributors

D.L. Arnold, Ph.D.
HPB, Health and Welfare Canada
Ottawa, Canada

J.L. Emerson, D.V.M., Ph.D.
The Coca-Cola Company
Atlanta, Georgia, U.S.A.

C.F. Hollander, M.D., Ph.D.
Institute for Experimental
   Gerontology TNO
Rijswijk, Netherlands

D.L. Knook, Ph.D.
Institute for Experimental
   Gerontology, TNO
Rijswijk, Netherlands

R. Kroes, D.V.M., Ph.D.
Institute CIVO Toxicology and
   Nutrition TNO
Zeist, Netherlands

D.N. McMartin, D.V.M., Ph.D.
Ciba-Geigy Corporation
Summit, New Jersey, U.S.A.

F.W. Oehme, D.V.M., Ph.D.
Kansas State University
Manhattan, Kansas, U.S.A.

P. Olsen, D.V.M., Ph.D.
National Food Institute
Soborg, Denmark

J. Sugar, M.D.
Research Institute of Oncopathology
Budapest, Hungary

C.F.A. van Bezooijen, Ph.D.
Institute of the Organization for
   Health Research TNO
Rijswijk, Netherlands

Acknowledgments

The authors wish to thank Carol L. Holliday for her assistance in preparation of this monograph.

Contents

I. Introduction

Age-associated changes in morphology and physiology have been demonstrated in virtually every tissue of aging humans and animals. As examples, age-associated changes in humans have been reviewed for the cardiovascular system (Lakatta, 1979), respiratory system (Maunderly, 1979), kidney (Epstein, 1979), neuroendocrine system (Finch, 1979) and physiological functions (Shock, 1979). Animals are also affected by aging (Finch, 1976; Hollander, 1970; Burek, 1978).

Rodents, the most commonly used experimental animals for chronic toxicity and carcinogenicity studies, like humans, develop many age-associated changes which have an impact on organ function and physiology. Such age-associated alterations in rodents take on increased importance because of the impact they can have on the results of long-term toxicity and carcinogenicity studies. Many age-associated lesions, both tumor and non-tumor, increase in severity, incidence or even total number per animal. As these lesions increase in number or become more severe, it is progressively more difficult to separate a toxic effect or early neoplastic changes from the normally occurring geriatric diseases, or to evaluate induced chemical changes that may be superimposed on the aging process.

The problem was not encountered in the 1950's and 1960's because it was unusual if the rodents on a long-term study survived much beyond 15 to 18 months. However, improvements in laboratory animal breeding, husbandry, facility design and better sources of commercially available rodents resulted in markedly improved survival. Increased longevity of rodents, coupled with the fact that the geriatric human population represents a steadily increasing percentage of the human population, has increased the need for a better understanding of the effects of chemicals on the geriatric age group.

A related problem concerns the duration of toxicity studies. Many guidelines for chronic testing are suggesting rodents should be maintained on test for longer than the traditional 18 months for mice and 24 months for rats, and some guidelines have stipulated either a specific time period or termination point based on the percentage of animals surviving in the various groups. There has been no good scientific rationale for extending the studies other than the fact that the animals survive longer.

Little information is available concerning the advantages and disadvantages of conducting toxicity tests that exceed 24 months.

This monograph will consider the physiological and pathological changes that occur in the aging rodent. Factors that may have an impact on the choice of duration for long-term rodent studies with a view to providing information to aid in establishing useful guidelines will be considered.

To address these issues, a number of factors will be reviewed and evaluated. These include the following:

1. The types of long-term studies that have been conducted in the past and those that may be undertaken in the future.

2. Considerations in the design and conduct of long-term toxicity studies.

3. How age-associated diseases complicate long-term studies.

4. Effects of aging on drug metabolism.

5. Cost of long-term studies.

6. Areas in need of future research.

II. Types of Long-Term Tests

A long-term toxicity study can be defined in several ways, but generally it is a study of several months to several years duration and usually involves rodents. This could include studies of three-months duration or longer. However, studies of approximately 3 months in length are often referred to as subchronic toxicity studies.

There are a number of other studies that can be included in the definition of long-term. For example, fertility and reproduction studies can be conducted over a period of several months or even several years in the case of multiple generation studies. Likewise, some teratology studies involve retention of offspring to maturity and subsequent breeding to permit evaluation of possible teratogenic effects in the second generation. Cytogenetic testing may be conducted on cells from animals treated for a prolonged period of time.

In order to provide a working definition for this monograph, studies of six months or less are excluded and long-term or chronic toxicity studies are defined as those toxicity tests that are of approximately 6 months duration or longer. Using this definition there are two main types of long-term toxicity studies. The first are the chronic toxicity tests and the second oncogenicity tests. It is possible to conduct each of these two tests separately or conduct one test which addresses both the chronic toxicity and oncogenicity question. The objective of such long-term studies is to evaluate and to characterize the effects produced by compounds when repeatedly administered to experimental animals over a period of months or years. The administration of the test substance may be on a daily basis as is common for all gavage, water and dietary studies or may be on an intermittent basis such as by the inhalation route with usual exposures of 6 hours/day, 5 days/week.

Several factors may influence the duration of long-term studies. Among these is the species of animals used, which could include monkeys, dogs, cats, rabbits or rodents. Only rarely are non-rodent species maintained on long-term toxicity studies to the point where their respective geriatric diseases actually impact on the conduct or interpretation of the studies. This is because they are too long-lived and the cost of lifetime studies with these animals would be prohibitive. Rodents are most commonly used and as a result, the major portion of this monograph discusses long-term toxicity studies that utilize rodents as the test species.

III. Factors Related to the Aging Process that Influence the Design and Conduct of Long-Term Rodent Studies

1. Introduction

Many factors should be considered when designing any rodent toxicity study. (These are outlined in the preceding document, "The Selection of Doses in Chronic Toxicity/Carcino genicity Studies" and a document prepared by the Institute of Laboratory Animal Resources (Committee on Long-Term Holding of Laboratory Rodents, 1976). The factors include species, strain or stock, sex, husbandry conditions (i.e., temperature, humidity, caging), nutrition, background of infectious and other diseases, historical tumor incidence, randomization procedures, test material, route, dose, and the need for interim kills during the study.

2. Species or Strain

The selection of the species and the strain or stock could impact on the results of a long-term study. Rats, mice, and hamsters can be conveniently housed in large numbers, thus providing greater numbers of animals for statistical evaluation of the data obtained. Because of physiologic peculiarities, the rat is sometimes the species of choice. The rat cannot vomit and emetic agents can be tested at higher dose levels in this species. The rat is also an obligant nasal breather and, hence, vapors, gases and other atmospheric contaminants that damage the mucosal lining of the nares and turbinates can be detected in inhalation studies using this species.

The species and strain of animal can determine the spontaneous disease background and can influence survival. If a relatively short-lived mouse strain such as the AKR is chosen, then it is unlikely good quality two-year data would be obtained since most of the animals would be dead prior to the 24 month terminal sacrifice. Although mice such as the B6C3Fl have a relatively high incidence of liver nodules and lymphosarcoma, they also have a high rate of survival: their 50% survival approaches 28-30 months of age. Likewise, rat strains have different survival rates. The 50% survival for most strains and stocks of rats is now in the range of 27-30 months. A measure of the improvement in longevity is seen with the commonly used Fisher 344. Several years ago the strain was considered to be relatively short-lived with a mean survival of about 14 months. Later the mean survival was reported to be around 22 months and currently the Fisher 344 is considered to be a long-lived rat strain with a mean survival of nearly 30 months.

3. Interim Sacrifices

Current guidelines recommend that the design of a long-term study include interim sacrifices. The principle reason for this is to permit thorough assessment of any toxic effects and to aid in defining their pathogenesis. Interim kills are also useful to help evaluate early stages in the tumor formation process. These have been scheduled at various times during long-term rodent studies. The most common perhaps, is a single interim sacrifice at 12 months, which is half-way through the study. Interim sacrifices at 6 and 12 months, or at 6, 12 and 18 months during a long-term rodent study are also employed. Recently the National Toxicology Program (NTP) in the U.S.A. has recommended a 15 month interim sacrifice for their long-term bioassay programs. The number of interim sacrifices and the times chosen is a decision that will probably vary depending upon the study and the type of data an investigator wishes to obtain. Such information is particularly important for the evaluation of chronic toxicity during the long-term studies.

4. Caging, Rooms and Route of Dosing

Caging is an important consideration because in long-term studies it is usually recommended that only one or two animals be housed per cage. This requires more cage resources and perhaps more rooms during the conduct of the long-term studies thereby increasing the cost of the study substantially. It is important with mice and hamsters to house males singly because of fighting which can confound interpretation of study results.

Ideally only one room per study and per species should be used. However, it does mean that the room will be unavailable for other uses for the duration of the study. Even though mortality may occur in a study and the numbers of animals in a given room may become relatively small, a second study should not be initiated in that same room until the first study has been terminated.

Other considerations in chronic study design include the route of administration. Dosing by gavage provides an accurate assessment of the dose administered and is practical for short-term studies. It is the preferred method if the test chemical must be given by the oral route and if it is highly volatile. The degree of stability may dictate dosing by gavage. However, for longer term studies it is usually simpler and more convenient to dose animals by way of feed or water. The route of exposure in animals should correspond to that in the human population.

5. Importance of Baseline Pathology Data

The background incidence of pathologic alterations and baseline chemistry and hematology data are important considerations in choosing an animal species and a strain or stock. Probably the most important single factor in the selection of the species of choice is the available historical background of pathologic alterations. Any increased incidence of a disease process that appears to be induced by a chemical should be appraised in the light of concurrent and historical control data. The historical data that may be available from the laboratory in which the study was conducted is particularly relevant but historical controls from other laboratories should also be taken into account. Unless there is good scientific data to the contrary, the chosen species and strain or stock should be ones for which the given laboratory has historical control data.

Detailed information on longevity is available for rats and mice (Storer, 1966; Burek, 1978; Coleman *et al.*, 1977; Gsell, 1964; Schlettwein-Gsell, 1970). These authors indicate that the 50% survival rate for most strains and stocks of rats and mice is in the range of 26 to 30 months. The 50% survival rate can be used as an indicator of population aging (Burek and Hollander, 1980). It can be used to determine if a population has reached the age where age-related mortality (i.e., related to old age or senescence) can be expected to rapidly increase.

This is illustrated in Figure 1 showing a typical rodent survival curve. When a two-year study is terminated, rodents are of an age where age-related mortality is rapid. By this time, approximately one half of the rodents have been treated for their complete life span and the survivors at 2 years are 26 months old and have been treated for the majority of their life spans.

The common lesions of rats and mice have been well documented. Non-

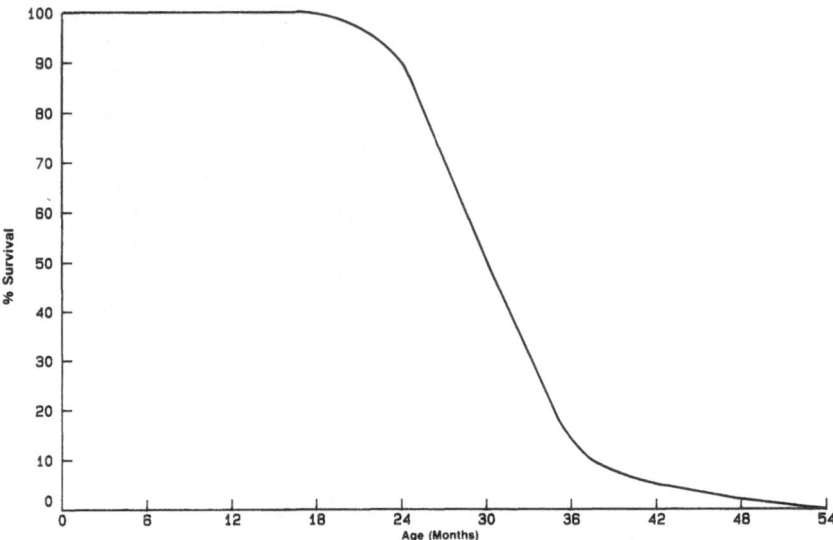

Figure 1. Typical rodent survival curve.

tumor pathology of rats has been reviewed (Berg and Simms, 1960, 1961, 1965; Berg, 1967; Boorman and Hollander, 1973; Bullock *et al.*, 1968; Burek, 1978; Cohen and Anver, 1976; Coleman *et al.*, 1977; Cotchin and Roe, 1967; Ribelin and McCoy, 1965; Anver and Cohen, 1979). Tumors have also been described (Boorman and Hollander, 1972, 1973; Burek and Hollander, 1977; Burek, 1978; Coleman *et al.*, 1977; Crain, 1958; Gilbert and Gillman, 1958; Roe, 1965; Thompson *et al.*, 1961; Turusov, 1973, 1976; Altman and Goodman, 1979). Likewise, the common lesions of aging mice have also been documented (Burek *et al.*, 1982).

In general, age-associated pathologic processes in rats and mice first begin to be recognized during the first year and increase in incidence and severity during the second year. The most rapid progression of age-associated lesions is from 24 months and beyond (Burek, 1978) so that rats and mice beyond 24 months of age have numerous neoplastic and nonneoplastic lesions. Figure 2 illustrates the average number of tumor and non-tumor lesions in a stock of Sprague-Dawley rats at various time periods. The average number of lesions by 24 months can exceed 30 per rat. In a F344 rat that has leukemia, the number of lesions can exceed 40 or 50 since many organs have leukemic infiltrates plus other geriatric diseases. The fact that most organs may have one or more age-associated lesions greatly complicates any evaluation for treatment-related effects. If the lesion has no human counterpart, extrapolation based on an increased incidence in the animal is tenuous. If the animal is afflicted with additional disease processes, then extrapolation to humans is

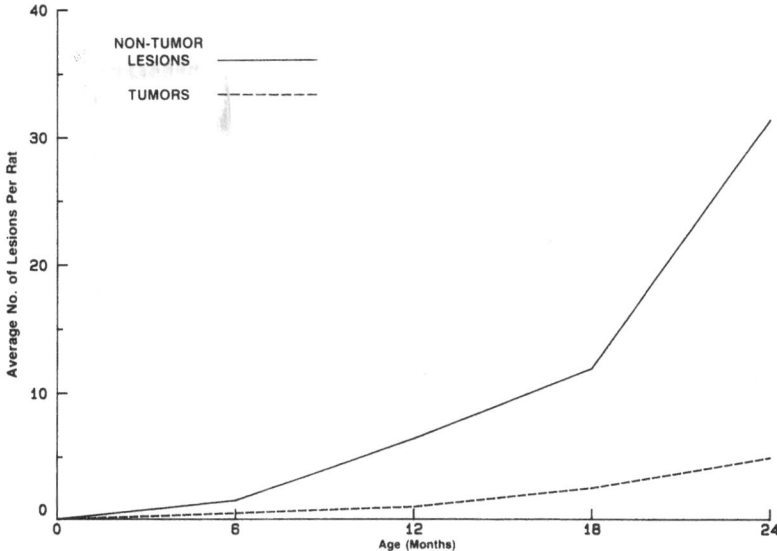

Figure 2. Average number of tumor and non-tumor lesions in rats at different ages. Data from a Sprague-Dawley rat strain.

inadvisable. The principle of employing healthy animals in toxicity studies should be adhered to for the duration of the study.

6. Diet

Variations in diet including quantity, quality, or both may significantly alter growth and longevity and may cause changes in neoplastic and nonneoplastic age-associated diseases. The importance of diet on longevity and age-associated pathology has been stressed (Berg and Simms, 1960, 1961 and 1965; Nolen, 1972; Ross et al., 1976; Ross, 1961; Ross and Bras, 1965, 1973). Cohen and Anver (1976) and Anver and Cohen (1979) have reviewed this topic in some depth.

Diets given to control and treated rodents are standardized, but treated rodents do not necessarily receive or utilize the same nutrients as controls. For example, compounds that affect food consumption or body weights can result in dose-related effects that are not necessarily a direct effect of the test material.

7. In-Life Evaluation of Animals

Many procedures may be employed to aid in the evaluation of the health of animals as a group and as individuals. There are a number of routine procedures that include observations regarding the normal physiological functions of eating, drinking, urinating and defecating; the animal's movement in the cage and its reaction to handling or to the housekeeping duties associated with its care (Arnold *et al.*, 1977; Fox *et al.*, 1977). If close observation suggests all these functions are normal, then the animal is likely in a state of good health. The need to have conscientious individuals who are familiar with the species under test attending to these duties, cannot be over-emphasized. Included in the routine tests are determinations of body weights and food consumption. These data help to establish dose levels for future studies and provide a reference point in order to evaluate the general health status of the animals. Body weight and food consumption is important for an evaluation of the health status of the individual and for the group as a whole. Animals that are affected by the test compound will usually show decreased body weight or food consumption in a dose-related manner. An infectious disease process that affects body weight may be identified by observation of a random change in food consumption and body weight. In this case these effects may be observed in all groups including controls. Other methods of evaluating animals clinically include an ophthalmoscopic examination. For rodents this may include a detailed evaluation of each animal at the initiation of the study and prior to the animals' sacrifice at the end of the study. Although not commonly used, a stethoscope can be a valuable tool in assessing respiratory disease in a rodent.

Blood and urine analyses provide useful information for evaluation of health status. The normal background of geriatric diseases in the animal will determine the expected variations in these particular tests. Likewise, the geriatric diseases that develop in the animal will influence the clinical evaluation of the animal and the diagnosis of the diseases made during the in-life portion of a study. The geriatric diseases can cause diagnostic problems in many organs and tissues, not just the primary target tissue.

8. Criteria for Euthanasia

It is important to minimize autolysis. To do this, animals must be euthanized. In making a decision to euthanize an animal, it is expected that good clinical judgement will be used. This involves studying the clinical history of the animal, making a clinical examination including the use of the diagnostic aids, and arriving at a diagnosis and prognosis regarding the animal's health status before deciding to terminate the animal (Arnold *et al.*, 1977). Each case should be well documented so that it is clearly evident why the animal was euthanized. In addition, such documentation may assist the pathologist in the selection of additional tissue samples and will facilitate study review and audits.

There are a number of clinical signs that serve to indicate that the prognosis is unfavorable and that euthanasia is probably advisable.

8.1 *Debility and Cachexia.* The persistent impairment of body functions such as urination and defecation may result in loss of strength and may be clinically manifested by weight loss, altered mobility and changes in behavioral responses to handling. In some cases this is a direct result of either organ dysfunction or tumors. Anorexia or adipsia, whether completely or partially sustained, are symptomatic of the associated debility. The extent of the impairment dictates the time frame within which a final decision regarding euthanasia must be made.

Debility, cachexia and changes in mobility may occur as a result of secondary complications. For example, the growth of a pituitary tumor may result in partial displacement and pressure on the brain thereby affecting mobility. Tumor growth, which presses on a nerve, can produce a localized paralysis. A large thymus tumor will impair respiratory function.

Symptoms of general ill health and malnutrition are characteristic of various disease conditions which are frequently associated with either rapid or gradual weight loss. It is inappropriate to treat any animal with a disease condition during a toxicological study, therefore, confirmation of a viral or bacterial disease state in a significant number of animals may require termination of the study.

8.2 *Pain.* Since treatment during a toxicological study is inappropriate, animals in obvious pain associated with accident or illness should be euthanized.

8.3 *Anorexia.* A mature rat which does not eat or drink can lose up to 40 grams of its body weight each day. The animal will not survive long under these conditions. Physical infirmities and occlusions of excretory processes should be appraised to determine if they are contributing to or causing the disease state. The decision regarding euthanasia for such cases should be made on a daily basis.

Partial and sustained anorexia is accompanied by a linear decline in body weight and a reduction in feed consumption (for example, 5-15 grams/day weight loss and approximately 5-10 grams of feed/day). This may be the initial clinical indication of a serious disease problem or may suggest malocclusion. The final decision to euthanize may be delayed for several days to ascertain whether the animal is able to attain a better health status. This decision is mainly based on the degree of debility. In the terminal stage, anorexia is usually complete.

Some specific disease conditions are considered in the next section. Diagnosis and a knowledge of the pathogenesis of these conditions as well as the manner in which the condition affects the animal's health may be used to determine an appropriate time of euthanasia in the affected animal.

IV. Age-Associated Diseases: How They Complicate Long-Term Toxicity Studies

1. Introduction

Age-associated diseases, as well as the entire aging process, can pose diagnostic problems because of the effect that they have in many organs and tissues (von Wittenau and Gans, 1981). The result of an age-associated disease process may not be confined to the target organ in question since effects in one organ may have ramifications in other organs and tissues. The geriatric disease may affect the clinical appearance of the animal and may alter organ and body weight determinations. To illustrate this, several examples will be given of specific disease problems or conditions which occur in an age-associated manner in a population of rodents. The incidence of the various lesions may vary with different strains and stocks of rodents. The lesions may complicate the interpretation of results from data obtained on long-term studies by altering an animal's response to a test compound.

2. Examples of Age-Associated Diseases that Complicate Long-Term Toxicity Studies

The following examples of age-associated diseases are not intended to be all inclusive, nor are they intended to represent all of the age-associated lesions observed in laboratory rodents.

2.1 *Chronic Progressive Glomerulonephropathy.* Chronic progressive glomerulonephropathy (CPG) is a spontaneously occurring disease in aging rats. The disease is strain and sex dependent, and the incidence and severity increases with age. Clinically, the animals affected by CPG appear relatively healthy until late in the stage of the disease process. Within the last few weeks of life they begin to undergo a rapid weight loss, often characterized by soiling in the perineal region and roughened hair coat. During this time food consumption of the individual animal decreases. Burek *et al.*, (1979), correlated the structural and functional changes in CPG in the rat. The earliest clinical chemistry value that was altered during the disease process was an increase in the serum phosphorus and a resulting reversal of the calcium to phosphorus ratio. At a later stage in the process, increases in the blood urea nitrogen (BUN) and creatinine, and increases in alkaline phosphatase, secondary to bone remodeling in the animals and decreases in total protein and albumin were observed. Increased protein and casts were seen in urines of such animals.

Gross and histopathologic findings in the kidneys have been well-documented and characterized. Grossly, the kidneys are enlarged, pale, often have a pitted cortical surface, and contain numerous cortical cysts. The histologic features have been reported by numerous authors (Andrew and Pruett, 1957, 1975; Elema and Arends, 1975; Gray, 1977; Gray et al., 1982; Hirokawa, 1975; Snell, 1967). The ultrastructural features have also been described (Couser and Stilmant, 1975; Gray et al., 1974; Hirokawa, 1975; Kraus and Cain, 1974; Arakaw, 1970; Arakaw and Tokunaga, 1972), and immunofluorescent studies have been performed (Bolten et al., 1976; Couser and Stilmant, 1975, 1976; Hirokawa, 1975).

The extra renal pathology that occurs in rats dying from CPG includes enlarged parathyroid glands due to secondary renal hyperplasia. Pale streaks in areas in a number of tissues including the heart, stomach and cecum, occur because of mineralization and degeneration within these tissues. Blood vessels have a loss of normal elasticity and contain pale streaks due to mineralization. Lungs are very often mottled and moist as a result of edema, hemmorhage and calcification. The bone undergoes fibrous osteodystrophy secondary to the renal disease (Burek et al., 1979; Itakura et al., 1977; Snell, 1967). It is apparent that many other organs are involved to some degree, either directly or indirectly with the disease process in the kidney.

When groups of animals are evaluated, CPG may be increased or decreased in a dose-related manner in groups of animals. Quite often the degree or incidence of CPG is reduced in the treated or exposed animals compared to their respective controls. A cause for this change is not always apparent, however the nutritional status of the animal can affect the degree of CPG. Lowering the protein or decreasing the caloric intake of a rat during its lifetime can greatly reduce the onset and severity of CPG. If dosing the animal affects the food consumption and body weight, then changes in CPG might be expected. Some strains or stocks of rats have a very high incidence of this disease, which can result in increased mortality and reduced survival. Virtually 100% of some stocks of rats of Sprague-Dawley origin have CPG in varying degrees of severity. Such a condition can interfere with the interpretation of chemically induced low grade chronic toxic effects in the kidneys as well as in other tissues. It is also likely that the degree of CPG could affect compounds that are either metabolized or excreted in the kidney and could thereby alter the toxicity or carcinogenicity of a compound.

2.2 *Leukemia in Fisher 344 Rats.* Leukemia is common in the Fisher 344 rat (Altman and Goodman, 1979; Moloney, et al., 1970). Like chronic renal disease, leukemia can have profound effects on many parameters. Clinically, animals with leukemia may show a slow or gradual weight loss and decrease in food consumption. They may have roughened hair coats and a slow wasting condition of the body. Soiling in the perineal region and development of icterus, or yellowish discoloration of the mucous membranes and extremities may occur late in the course of the disease. Leukemia can have profound effects on the clinical chemistry and hematology data obtained from animals during the in-life portion of the study. Animals with generalized leukemia very often have elevated serum liver enzymes and elevated BUN, values as well as alterations in hematologic values due to the circulating tumor cells. Anemia is another complicating factor of this disease. Grossly and histologically, nearly all organs may be affected by the leukemic process. Livers may be severely infiltrated by tumor cells, as may be the case for kidney, lung, brain and other tissues. Very often the spleen appears to be the target tissue and is extremely enlarged due to the infiltration of tumor cells. Obviously, such widespread disseminated tumor can affect the body weight, individual organ weights, blood data, and make it difficult to evaluate other tumor and non-tumor pathology. Hence data from these animals should not be included in tabulations of mean data such as body and organ weights, blood values and urinalysis data.

The incidence of leukemia is highly variable in the Fisher 344 rat. In some strains, the incidence varies from l0-25% after two years and up to 40 or even 50% at 30 months of age. Animals affected with leukemia are of little value for evaluating chronic toxic or carcinogenic effects that may have been produced by a test compound. When the incidence of a geriatric disease reaches such high proportions with advancing age, the advisability of continuing studies past 24 months should be seriously questioned.

2.3 *Mammary Tumors.* Mammary tumors occur in most stocks and strains of rats, but particularly in certain stocks of Sprague-Dawley rats, where the incidence may exceed 80% of all females on a two-year study. Usually such tumors are benign and are characteristically diagnosed as fibroadenomas. Although benign, such tumors may increase in size, become massive, are often traumatized, and interfere with locomotion. The end result is often intermittent bleeding, secondary anemia, extramedullary hematopoiesis in several tissues, and even eventual death due to blood loss. On long-term studies the occurrence and progression of these tumors should be documented over the course of the study.

2.4 *Peripheral Nerve Degeneration.* Age-associated peripheral nerve degeneration is a relatively common geriatric disease which occurs in many different strains and stocks of rats (Burek *et al.*, 1976; van Steenis and Kroes, 1971). The incidence of the disease is highly variable but may affect as many as 80% of some old rats (Burek, 1978). In the mild form of the disease there is little to be observed clinically and the disease or lesions are recognized only on the histopathologic examination. However the disease may progress and eventually lead to posterior paresis and paralysis. Animals may become anuric and develop secondary uremia and die. This condition can be a complicating factor on long-term studies particularly with test compounds that cause peripheral neuropathy such as n-butyl ketone, n-hexane or acrylamide. In all of these cases it is important to differentiate the age-associated lesions from induced lesions. Animal strains with a high background of this condition are unsuitable subjects for long-term tests on compounds that cause peripheral neuropathy.

2.5 *Amyloidosis*. Amyloidosis is a fairly common age-associated lesion in certain strains of mice and hamsters. Clinically, an animal with amyloidosis may appear only as a sick animal which may show soiling in the perineal region due to excess urination. However in severe forms, where liver and kidneys are both affected, subcutaneous edema may be present and ascites may result in abdominal distention. Amyloidosis may affect urine, hematology and clinical chemistry values, and in particular total protein may be decreased in the blood. Gross and histopathologic examination reveals amyloid deposits in organs such as the spleen, thyroid, liver, adrenals, kidneys, intestinal tract and other sites as well. Like chronic progressive glomerulonephropathy, amyloid may be either increased or decreased in the experimental groups compared to the controls. The cause for this is not always apparent but nutrition may play a role. When the liver and kidneys are severely affected many clinical chemistry measurements such as transaminase and BUN values are secondarily altered.

2.6 *Pituitary Tumors*. Pituitary tumors occur in both rats and mice. The incidence may vary from about 20% to as high as 80 or 90% in aging rats of some strains. Two main effects are secondary to the pituitary tumors in rodents and these can be related either to the pressure changes caused by the expanding mass within the calvarium, or changes secondary to hormonal factors. Clinically, pituitary tumors may be occult or animals may manifest signs including weight loss and a general decrease in activity, with animals often sitting hunched in the corner of the cage. They may have bulging of the eyes, prophyrin-like pigment around the eyes and nose, head tilts, proliferation of mammary tissue, increased mammary tumors and galactocele formation. Galactocele formation in male rats is pathognomonic for a pituitary tumor.

2.7 *Interstitial Cell Tumors in Fisher 344 Rats*. Interstitial cell hyperplasia and tumor formation are common in Fisher 344 rats (Jacobs and Huseby, 1967; Coleman, *et al.*, 1977). They are common by 12 months of age and by 24 months of age virtually 100% of survivors have developed single or multiple interstitial cell tumors. The lesions are often of varying sizes. There is an associated atrophy, which may be a spontaneous geriatric atrophy or secondary to the expanding tumor mass from the interstitial cells. Such spontaneous lesions clearly alter the testicle and make it impossible to evaluate drug or chemically induced testicular changes in this rat strain. As a result, the Fisher 344 rat is not an appropriate species to use to test compounds that could affect the testicle.

2.8 *Chronic Foot Problems.* Animals housed in wire-bottom cages for long periods of time can develop chronic foot problems due to irritation. The foot problems may manifest themselves as small wart-like growths on one or more feet. There may be generalized swelling of the affected foot that may cause problems in locomotion. Such lesions are often ignored by the attendants and pose no serious problem to the health or well being of the animal on the long-term study. On the other hand, some animals do develop more extensive foot problems which might include ulceration and irritation to the feet themselves. Chronic bleeding problems and secondary infection may occur which may lead to anemia. Enlargement of inguinal and auxillary lymph nodes may be seen. Therefore, the caging may influence the survivability and health and well-being of animals on the long-term studies and pose another complicating factor that does not occur to a significant degree in short-term studies. The use of shoe-box cages eliminates this problem.

2.9 *Overgrown Incisor Teeth.* Incisor teeth of rodents tend to continue to grow with age and are normally worn down by the eating and feeding process. If there is malocclusion, the incisor teeth may overgrow so that the animals can no longer eat properly. The problem becomes even more pronounced when long-term dietary studies are conducted with finely mashed or finely ground feed, since the finely ground feed is not sufficiently abrasive to wear the teeth down in a normal fashion. Overgrown teeth may result in ulcerations, particularly caused by lower teeth growing up behind the upper teeth resulting in secondary ulcerations and inflammation. The end result is chronic weight loss secondary to the tooth problems and secondary infections within the ulcerated portions of the mouth. Secondary ulcerative and inflammatory lesions may lead to changes in the hematological parameters. The animals begin to lose weight and eventually starve to death if the condition is uncorrected by trimming the teeth.

2.10 *Discussion.* The above examples of conditions that affect animals on long-term studies serve to illustrate that age-associated geriatric diseases can affect the animals in many ways, including their clinical appearance, clinical chemistry values, hematology values, and the urinalysis data. It is important to know the historical background incidence of such conditions and to appreciate how the diseases and their sequelae can confuse and complicate the gross and histopathologic evaluation of tissues.

Although the diseases may primarily affect a principal organ, the development of lesions in other organs commonly follows. In addition, the disease processes may render the animal more susceptible to secondary infections. Under such conditions, attempts to attribute observed lesions to toxicity of a test chemical is a difficult and questionable practice.

It is clear that the longer the animals live, the greater the probability that these diseases will complicate the outcome of a study. This in turn renders an appraisal of the study more difficult and tenuous, with meaningful extrapolation of the findings to humans highly questionable.

V. Effect of Aging on Drug Metabolism

1. Introduction

Drug response variations occur in humans and animals. Individual drug response variations might be due to differences in drug pharmacokinetics and metabolism and may depend on both the drug and population selected for investigation.

A clearer understanding of the causes of differences in the rate of drug elimination is necessary. Over the past several years, animal studies indicate that the causes can be subdivided into external environmental, internal environmental and pharmacological (Vesell, 1980). Included in the internal environmental variables are genetic constitution, disease, sex and age. External environmental variables include diet, smoking, alcohol intake, etc. Pharmacological variables include the route of drug elimination and drug interactions. These factors can determine how any drug is tolerated by a patient and can affect the safety of the compound.

These factors may have a major impact on the design and results obtained from long-term animal studies since old and young rodents may or may not react similarly to xenobiotics. Recent reviews, which deal primarily with the increased incidence of adverse drug reactions in geriatric human patients, suggest that age may have an effect (Gillette, 1979; Richey and Bender, 1977; Vestal, 1978; Schmucker, 1979) on how drugs are handled by the body. Since most dosages used in chronic tests are based on the response of young animals during shorter (usually 90-day) periods, it is important these questions be addressed.

This portion of the monograph will review the effects of age on toxicity, xenobiotic metabolism and other pharmacokinetic measurements.

Special emphasis will be placed on age changes in the liver because of the importance of this organ in detoxification and drug metabolism.

2. *In Vivo* Demonstrations of Aging Effects on Toxicity

Few studies with the stated purpose of evaluating age effects on histological damage produced by the administration of a chemical to an animal have been reported. Horita *et al.* (1980) gave 6-aminonicotinamide (6-AN) daily to male rats aged 3, 15, 20 and 25 months for 3, 5, 7 or 14 days. The youngest rats developed clinical signs of central nervous system dysfunction by day 3 and histologic brain lesions by days 5 and 7, however, these signs and lesions had disappeared by day 14. In contrast, signs and lesions persisted in the older rats and became progressively worse with increasing age. The lesions produced by 6-AN consisted of a spongy state of the gray matter and neuronal chromatolysis similar to that seen in Creutzfeldt-Jakob disease.

High doses of D-galactosamine caused hepatic necrosis probably by producing an acute deficiency of uridine triphosphate below a threshold of 30% of normal. The amount of hepatic necrosis produced by a single administration of this compound was found by Platt et al. (1978) to be greater in 30-month-old than in 6-week-old female SIV rats. Prednisolone protected against damage in the younger but not the older rats. Damage was detected morphologically and also by release of cytoplasmic and hepatic lysosomal enzymes into plasma.

Jones et al. (1973) fed clioquinol in a maize diet to rats for over 125 weeks and found that the rats fed clioquinol developed a much more severe neuropathy in old age than did rats fed only a maize diet (for 123 weeks or less). Other investigators (Hess et al., 1972) had not been able to produce a neuropathy in rats during a previous subchronic (90-day) study. Jones et al. (1973) concluded that clioquinol can accentuate the neuropathy commonly seen in old rats.

Several investigators who used drug administration to investigate a gerontological problem unexpectedly found that these compounds were more toxic to older animals. For example, Massie et al. (1980) found that daily oral administration of phenytoin elevated serum copper and ceruloplasmin concentrations less in old (654-746 days) male C57BL/6J mice than in young (136-199 days) and middle-aged (427-448 days) animals. However, mortality in the old group was so high that phenytoin could be given for only four days in contrast to the 14-day treatment received by younger mice. Likewise, Greenberg and Weiss (1979), while showing that old rats have an impaired ability to increase beta receptor density in their brains after reserpine injections, found that the drug was more toxic to older animals. Three-month-old rats could tolerate three daily doses of 8 mol/kg reserpine, but 50 to 75% of 24-month-old rats died after receiving only two daily doses of 2 or 4 mol/kg. Kao and Hudson (1980) used four daily injections of phenobarbitone to induce the hepatic drug metabolizing system in 10 and 100-week-old F344 rats. They commented that a dosage, which was satisfactory in younger rats, produced much heavier sedation and even death in their older rats. McMartin et al. (1980) similarly found that a dose of phenobarbital used routinely for hepatic enzyme induction in young adult rats was lethal to older ones.

Caffeine and ethanol produce different toxicity in young and middle-aged animals. Peters and Boyd (1967) administered 185 mg/kg caffeine daily, a dose slightly higher than the LD_{50}, to male and female rats aged 1.5, 2.5,

4.5 and 12 months. Caffeine was found to be more toxic to the oldest rats, killing 69 and 77% of the females and males respectively, as compared to 0 to 33% mortality in any other age group. In this connection, Latini *et al.* (1980) found that the elimination of caffeine was slower in 12-month-old Sprague-Dawley rats ($t_{1/2}$ = 332 min.) than in 40-day-old rats ($t_{1/2}$ = 120 min.)

Wiberg *et al.* (1970) reported that the acute LD_{50} of ethanol was also lower in 10 to 12-month-old male Wistar rats than in 3 to 4-month-old animals. Delayed clearance of ethanol from blood and brain and slower metabolism as measured *in vitro* with liver slices contributed to the increased toxicity in the older animals. Similarly, Abel (1978) showed that ethanol caused 12 to 13-month-old female C57BL/6J mice to sleep longer than younger (2-3 months) animals.

The toxicity of ethanol may continue to increase as the animal ages if, as postulated by Sun and Samorajski (1975), the *in vitro* inhibition of (Na^+ + K^+)-ATPase activity in brain synaptosomes is an indicator of *in vivo* effects. They showed that this enzyme became more susceptible to ethanol inhibition with increasing age of the mouse. Male C57BL/10 mice aged 3, 8 and 26-29 months were used. Recent findings by Ritzmann and Springer (1980) also suggest that old C57BL/6 mice were more susceptible to central nervous system effects elicited by ethanol. Their 24-month-old mice had lower ethanol concentrations in their brain at the time the righting response was lost than did animals aged 6 and 12 months. Old mice also had slower uptake of ethanol into blood and brain after intraperitoneal injection and slower clearance from blood.

3. Effects of Aging on Pharmacokinetics in Rodents

The toxicity of a compound is related to the concentration that reaches its target tissue which, in turn, is controlled by absorption, protein binding, metabolism and excretion.

3.1 *Absorption.* Available reports concerning the effect of aging on intestinal absorption were limited to those dealing with glucose, vitamin A and five amino acids. Glucose absorption from the small intestine lumen increased during the first ten months but remained constant thereafter until at least 32 months in CD rats (Klimas, 1968).

In contrast, 6-deoxy-D-glucose absorption from the intestine of male and female C57BL/6 mice did not change between 29 days and 21 to 24 months. This compound is particularly useful because it is absorbed similarly to glucose but is not metabolized (Calingaert and Zorzoli, 1965). Intestinal absorption of vitamin A increased linearly from 25% at 1.5 months to 37% at 39 months in male Sprague-Dawley rats (Hollander and Morgan, 1979).

The *in vivo* intestinal absorption of lysine, arginine and proline increased between 12 and 25 or 27 months in female Wistar rats while the absorption of tryptophane and phenylalanine remained unaffected by aging. The age effects on the first two amino acids were apparent only at luminal concentrations of 5 mM or less (Penzes, 1974; Penzes and Boross, 1974).

3.2 *Plasma and Tissue Binding.* Alterations in the amount of drug or test compound that binds to plasma proteins can change the amount of agent that reaches its target tissue or is excreted since bound drug may not, for example, readily cross the blood-brain barrier or be filtered through the glomerulus. Changes in protein binding capacity will also result in changes in the hepatic clearance of drugs that are poorly absorbed by the liver.

Jones and Pardon (1980) found that the percentage of pentobarbitone bound to mouse plasma proteins did not change significantly between donor ages of 3 and 24 months. The protein binding of drugs in the blood is determined mainly by the serum albumin concentration. Accordingly, binding was found to correlate significantly with plasma albumin concentration and albumin was slightly decreased in the older mice. The albumin concentration in plasma was reported to be unchanged (de Leeuw-Israel, 1971), slightly lower (Pardon *et al.*, 1977) or significantly lower (Coleman, *et al.*, 1977), respectively, in old (RXU) F_1, BN/BI, and F344 male rats.

The degree of tissue binding or distribution of a compound into tissues other than plasma may also change with age. Klotz (1979) found that the elimination half-life of plasma diazepam in 18-month old Wistar rats was twice as long as in 6-month-old rats. He suggested that the slower elimination of this lipophilic drug was probably due to the increased adipose mass in the older rats. Metabolism was not determined. Conway *et al.* (1979) measured the *in vitro* binding of warfarin to homogenates of skeletal muscle, liver and kidney. Binding remained constant up to 360 days and then decreased to 59-73% of young adult values by 832 days of age. Plasma warfarin binding was unaffected by increasing age. They concluded that lowered tissue binding could increase the amount of drug in the body which is free to circulate.

4. Age and Hepatic Drug Metabolism

The liver, more so than any other organ, is responsible quantitatively and qualitatively for the metabolism of more xenobiotics. Because of this, special attention will be given to the effects of aging on its morphology, physiological chemistry and metabolism of drugs.

4.1 Age-Related Changes in Liver Morphology

4.1.1 *Liver Weight.* Age-related changes in liver weight play an important role in the capacity of the liver to metabolize drugs or chemicals. Since the dose of a drug is usually based on body weight, the liver weight to body weight ratio is most relevant. Liver weight to body weight ratios can range from 2.0 to 5.0% in animals of the same age depending on the strain, sex and age of the animals used. Changes in the overall liver weight to body weight ratio with age are shown in Table I.

4.1.2 *Ploidy Status.* Ploidy is the state of the cell nucleus relating to the number of genomes present. A pronounced age-related change in liver morphology is the shift of the hepatocytes to a higher ploidy. This increase in polyploidy of rat hepatocytes with age is strain dependent. Although the pattern of the shift is mostly identical, that is a shift from mononuclear diploid via binuclear diploid to mononuclear tetraploid and via binuclear tetraploid to mononuclear octaploid, the time onset and the end of the ploidy changes differ from strain to strain (van Bezooijen, 1978). Generally, it can be stated that the most pronounced changes in the ploidy state in rats occur during the first year of life. Changes in the ploidy of the hepatocytes in mice are more spectacular. They continue to the age of at least 28 months and ploidy values of 16 and 32 N are quite common (Shima and Sugahara, 1976).

It is possible that age changes in the metabolism of drugs and other chemical compounds by the liver *in vivo* are partly attributable to age-related changes in the ploidy state of the hepatocytes. Assuming that a mononuclear diploid

Table I. Changes in Liver Weight to Body Weight Ratio with Age

Species	Sex	Strain	Liver weight/ Body weight ratio[a]	Reference
Rat	F	Wistar	−	Kato & Takanaka, 1968a
Rat	M	Wistar	=	Kitani et al., 1978
Rat	M	Wistar	−	Ali et al., 1979
Rat	M	Wistar	=	McMartin et al., 1980
Rat	F	RU	=	de Leeuw-Israel, 1971
Rat	F	WAG/Rij	=	van Bezooijen & Knook, 1978
Rat	F	WAG/Rij	−	Kitani et al., 1982
Rat	M	WAG/Rij	−	Kitani et al., 1982
Rat	F	BN/Bi 3–12 mo.	−	Kitani et al., 1982
		3–24 & 30	=	Kitani et al., 1982
Mouse	M	NIH White Swiss	=	Jones, 1967
Mouse	F	NIH White Swiss	=	Jones, 1967

[a] − denotes decrease with age; = denotes no change with age.

cell has less volume than a binuclear diploid or a mononuclear tetraploid cell (which have less volume than a binuclear tetraploid or mononuclear octaploid cell), the number of hepatocytes per unit liver volume will decrease with age. Consequently, the amount of cell surface will also decrease with age. Since drugs and other compounds are transported across the hepatocyte membrane and the sinusoidal membrane area involved in drug uptake may be relatively decreased, the rate of uptake may be influenced by the observed increase in polyploidy of the hepatocytes.

4.1.3 *Smooth Endoplasmic Reticulum.* The smooth endoplasmic reticulum (SER) is the intracellular structure directly responsible for the hepatic capacity to metabolize drugs or chemicals. Data concerning age related changes in the amount of SER in rats are quite conflicting. Pieri *et al.* (1975) observed an increase in the cytoplasmic volume occupied by the SER between 12 and 27 months. However, Schmucker *et al.* (1977) found a decrease in the amount of SER between 10 and 30 months. These discrepancies might be due to differences in the methods, strain, and sex of the rats employed by the two groups. Pieri *et al.* (1975) used the immersion fixation method and female Wistar rats. Schmucker *et al.* (1977) used the preferable perfusion fixation method and male Fischer 344 rats. A study performed by Meihuizen and Blansjaar (1980) using the perfusion fixation method and female WAG/Rij rats revealed an increase in the cytoplasmic volume occupied by the SER between 3 and 35 months of age. Pieri *et al.* (1978) also studied age-related changes in the SER in mouse

Table II. Common Spontaneous Nonneoplastic Age-Related Liver Lesions in Various Rat Strains

Tumor[a]	Strain	Sex	Age (mos.)	Frequency[b] (%)	Reference
Foci or areas of cellular alteration	WAG/Rij	M	24[c]	36	Burek, 1978
Foci or areas of cellular alteration	WAG/Rij	F	32[c]	84	Burek, 1978
Altered cell foci	Wistar	M	31–36[d]	84	McMartin *et al.*, 1980
Bile duct hyperplasia	Fischer	M	<25[d]	98	Coleman *et al.*, 1977
Bile duct cysts	BN/Bi	M	32[c]	26	Burek, 1978
Bile duct cysts	BN/Bi	F	33[c]	55	Burek, 1978
Dilated common bile ducts	WAG/Rij	M	30[c]	<20	Kitani *et al.*, 1982
Hepatic telangiectasis	WI	F	18[d]	50	Jones, 1967b
Hepatic telangiectasis	WI	M	18[d]	60	Jones, 1967b

[a] Only those lesions which occurred with a prevalence of 20% or more are included.
[b] Percentage of rats in which the lesion has been observed.
[c] Mean age when killed moribund.
[d] Age at interim kill.

liver; no significant changes between 12 and 24 months of age were observed. It appears that changes in the SER with age are species, strain and sex dependent. Therefore, it is difficult to generalize about the influence of changes in the SER with age on the capacity of the liver to metabolize drugs and chemicals.

4.1.4 *Histopathology.* In addition to general aging changes in liver morphology, specific histopathological changes occur in the livers of old rats. Spontaneous lesions observed in the liver of various rat strains are shown in Table II. Such liver lesions occurring in mice are shown in Table III. Only those lesions which occurred with a prevalence of 20% or more are included.

It is clear from the histopathological data presented in these tables that rat and mouse strains differ considerably in the type and frequency of liver lesions observed. The age-associated lesions could influence the capacity of the liver to metabolize xenobiotics. These conditions should be taken into account when studying the changes in the capacity of the liver to metabolize drugs or other chemical compounds and in long-term toxicity studies.

Table III. Common Spontaneous Neoplastic and Nonneoplastic Age-Related Liver Lesions in Various Mouse Strains

Tumor[a]	Strain	Sex	Age (mos.)	Frequency[b] (%)	Reference
"Hepatomas"	C3HeB/Da	F	24[c]	58	Deringer, 1956
"Hepatomas"	CBA/J	M		65	Storer, 1966
"Hepatomas"	CF-1	M	30[c]	34	Tomatis et al., 1974
"Hepatomas"	C3Hf	M	14[c]	31	Den Engelse et al., 1974
"Hepatomas"	CBA	M	30[c]	100	Sharp et al., 1976
"Hepatomas"	CF-1	M	28[c]	27	Ponomarkov & Tomatis, 1976
"Hepatomas"	SWJ/Jac	M	21[c]	63	Jacobs & Dieter, 1978
Liver cell neoplasms	C₃H-A^{vy}fB	M	15[c]	83	Ward & Vlahakis, 1978
Hepatocellular neoplasm type A	CBA	M	28[d]	23	Blankwater, 1978
Hepatic neoplasm (basophilic)	B6C3F1	M	18[c]	25	Hoover et al., 1980
Amyloidosis	C57B1/Ka	M	23[d]	83	Blankwater, 1978
Amyloidosis	C57B1/Ka	F	20[d]	73	Blankwater, 1978
Ischemic liver cell necrosis	NZB	M	17[d]	26	Blankwater, 1978
Ischemic liver cell necrosis	NZB	F	14[d]	33	Blankwater, 1978

[a] Only those lesions which occurred with a prevalence of 20% or more are included.
[b] Percentage of rats in which the lesion has been observed.
[c] Age at interim kill.
[d] Mean age when killed moribund.

4.2 *Age-Related Changes in Liver Physiology*

4.2.1 *Possible Contribution of Nonparenchymal Liver Cells.* Age-related changes in liver physiology are caused not only by intrinsic changes in the hepatocytes but also can be due to extrahepatic factors such as neurological, endocrinological and circulatory phenomena. The mammalian liver consists of various cell types, which can be divided into two principle groups: parenchymal cells (hepatocytes) and nonparenchymal cells. The latter population consists mainly of endothelial and Kupffer cells, both of which can be considered as major components of the reticuloendothelial system (Praaning-van Dalen *et al.*, 1981). The functional capacity of the reticuloendothelial system, as determined by the clearance rate of particulate material from the bloodstream, was reported to decline with age in both mice (Aoki *et al.*, 1965; Jaroslow and Larrick, 1973) and rats (Bilder, 1975). However, most of these studies did not include truly senescent animals and, therefore, little is known about the function of the reticuloendothelial system in senescent animals (Brouwer and Knook, 1983). Moreover, other functions of the reticuloendothelial system that directly concern Kupffer and endothelial liver cells were not studied during aging (Brouwer and Knook, 1983). Aging studies on the functional capacity of purified Kupffer cells in maintenance culture have been performed only recently. Preliminary results indicate that neither the capacity of these cells to endocytose heat-aggregated colloidal albumin nor the intracellular degradation of this substrate are affected by the age of the donor rat (Brouwer and Knook, 1983). Biochemical studies focused mainly on lysosomal enzymes indicated no general age-related decline in enzyme activities in the two cell types (Knook and Sleyster, 1976, 1978).

In summary, little is known about the functional changes in sinusoidal liver cells during aging and their possible contribution to the physiological changes in the whole liver are difficult to estimate.

4.2.2 *Physiological Metabolism.* The liver plays an important role in carbohydrate, protein and lipid metabolism. Changes with age in these functions of the hepatocyte were recently reviewed: carbohydrate metabolism by Sanadi (1978), and protein metabolism by van Bezooijen (1978). Changes in the lipid metabolism were described in Section 5 of the volume, *Liver and Ageing - 1978* (Kitani, 1977).

4.2.2.1 *Protein and Albumin Metabolism.* Recent studies on age-related changes in protein synthesis in isolated rat hepatocytes reveal that the changes are strain and sex dependent. A decrease for female WAG/Rij rats (van Bezooijen, *et al.*, 1977), for female Sprague-Dawley (Ricca *et al.*, 1979) and for male Fischer rats (Coniglio *et al.*, 1979) was observed during the first year of life. However, no change in protein synthesis between 3 and 12 months of age was

found for male Sprague-Dawley (Viskup *et al.*, 1979), male WAG/Rij and female BN/Bi rats (van Bezooijen *et al.*, 1981). Between 12 and 18-24 months, no change in protein synthesis by isolated hepatocytes was observed for male and female WAG/Rij and female BN/Bi (van Bezooijen *et al.*, 1977, 1981), female Sprague-Dawley (Ricca *et al.*, 1979) or male Fischer rats (Coniglio *et al.*, 1979). However, in male Sprague-Dawley rats, a decrease in protein synthesis was found in this age period (Viskup *et al.*, 1979). In advanced age, a sharp increase in the protein synthesizing capacity was observed for female WAG/Rij (van Bezooijen *et al.*, 1977), male Fischer (Coniglio *et al.*, 1979), and male WAG/Rij and female BN/Bi rats (van Bezooijen *et al.*, 1981). From these results, it is likely that the sharp increase in protein synthesis in hepatocytes isolated from old rats is independent of strain and sex.

Albumin is important as a transport protein for anions, fatty acids and drugs. The influence of age on the capacity of isolated hepatocytes to synthesize albumin was studied for female WAG/Rij rats (van Bezooijen *et al.*, 1976). A decrease in albumin synthesis was observed between 3 and 24 months of age, followed by a sharp increase in late age.

The observed increase in albumin and protein synthesis in late age might be a mechanism by which the liver attempts to compensate for increased excretion of protein via the urine, increased proteolytic activity or the occurrence of altered, malfunctional proteins. This supposed compensational capacity may enable the liver to maintain the serum concentration of albumin constant with age.

4.2.2.2 Lipid Metabolism.

With respect to the age changes seen in lipid metabolism and their influences on drug metabolism, it can be speculated that competing reactions for cofactors necessary for fatty acid synthesis may play a role in determining the availability of reduced nicotinamide dinucleotide phosphate (NADPH) involved in the mixed functions oxidase system. We are not aware of studies on the effect of age on the competing reactions for cofactors.

4.2.2.3 Carbohydrate Metabolism.

Changes in carbohydrate metabolism with age can influence the capacity of the liver to metabolize drugs. For example, the generation of NADPH may be rate controlling in drug metabolism capacity, since the supply of this reduced cofactor is most important in the maintenance of the oxidation-reduction state of the NADP/NADPH couple. NADPH is generated by the pentose phosphate pathway in a series of reactions starting with glucose-6-phosphate and involving the enzymes glucose-6-phosphate dehydrogenase (G6PDH) and 6-phosphogluconate dehydrogenase (6PGDH). NADPH is also generated by a malate shuttle which involves the production of NADPH from malate via the malic enzyme. Results of studies in rats on changes in G6PDH activity with age are contradictory; no change (Webb and

Bailey, 1975) as well as an increase or a decrease (Wang and Mays, 1977) have been reported. An increase in G6PDH activity was observed with age in mice (Wilson, 1972; Webb and Bailey, 1975). No change with age was observed in the activity of the malic enzyme.

These data suggest that there may be no age-related decrease in NADPH production due to a decrease in energy supply via the pentose phosphate pathway or the malate shuttle.

4.3 *Hepatic Drug Metabolism.* Drugs are generally metabolized by the liver in two phases; the so-called Phase I and Phase II metabolism. Phase I metabolism comprises reactions in which lipophilic drugs are transformed by oxidation, hydrolyses and reductions. Phase II metabolism includes those reactions in which drugs or their Phase I metabolites are transformed to less lipophilic metabolites by conjugation with small endogenous molecules, e.g., glucuronic acid or glutathione.

Most drugs undergo oxidation as a Phase I reaction. This is catalyzed by the mixed function oxidase (MFO) system. This system has as important components a series of hemoproteins collectively known as cytochrome P450, cytochrome b_5 and a flavoprotein referred to as NADPH-cytochrome P-450 (or C) reductase. These components are localized in the smooth endoplasmic reticulum of the hepatocyte and appear after fractionation in the microsomal fraction. In Table IV, age-related changes in cytochrome P450 and NADPH-cytochrome c-reductase activities are reviewed. Most studies report a decrease with age in the cytochrome P-450 concentration and the NADPH-cytochrome c-reductase activity. However, some authors reported no age-related differences.

Table IV. The Effect of Age on Mixed Function Oxidase Activities

Species	Cytochrome P450[a]	NADPH-cytochrome c-reductase	Reference
Rat	−	−	Kato & Takanaka, 1968a,b
Rat		=	Adelman, 1971
Rat		−	Grinna & Barber, 1972
Rat		−	Gold & Widnell, 1974
Rat	=	−	Baird et al., 1975
Rat	=	=	Birnbaum & Baird, 1978a
Rat	−	=	Birnbaum & Baird, 1978b
Rat	−		Platt, 1977
Rat	−	−	Schmucker & Wang, 1980
Rat	−		Kao & Hudson, 1980
Rat	−	−	McMartin et al., 1980
Mouse	−		Stohs et al., 1980

[a] − denotes decrease with age; = denotes no change with age.

Birnbaum and Baird (1979) found that conjugation of styrene oxide by glutathione-S-transferase from rat and mouse livers was unchanged at 3, 12, and 24 months. Ali *et al.* (1979) determined that hepatic glucuronidation was decreased by either 9 or 24% (depending on the substrate used) as their rats aged from 8 to 30 months. They concluded that this change would unlikely be of great clinical significance.

Many investigators have studied the influence of age on several liver microsomal drug-metabolizing enzymes. Their data are summarized in Table V. Most enzyme activities decreased with age, with the exception of pyroxidal kinase and pyridoxamine-P oxidase which did not change. In contrast, an increase in activity was observed for epoxide hydrase.

A few studies have been performed concerning the effect of age on the *in vivo* metabolism of drugs. Results of these studies are reviewed in Table VI. Metabolizing capacity seems to be decreased with age in rats. In two out of three studies in mice, no change in the metabolizing capacity was found.

Some of the earliest studies on the effects of aging on drug metabolism used agents that were metabolized by the MFO system. In 1961, Verzar reported that about 60% as much hexobarbital was needed to anesthetize 29-32 month-old rats as was needed to produce a similar degree of narcosis in 4-5 month-

Table V. Changes in Drug Metabolizing Enzyme Activities with Age

Species	Enzyme	Change with age[a]	Reference
Rat	Hexobarbital hydroxylase	−	Kato & Takanaka, 1968a,b
Rat	Aminopyrine N-dimethylase	−	Kato & Takanaka, 1968a,b
Rat	Aniline hydroxylase	−	Kato & Takanaka, 1968a,b
Rat	Strychnine oxidase	−	Kato & Takanaka, 1968a,b
Rat	p-nitrobenzoic acid reductase	−	Kato & Takanaka, 1968a,b
Rat	p-dimethylaminobenzene reductase	−	Kato & Takanaka, 1968a,b
Rat	Zoxazolamine hydroxylase	−	Baird *et al.*, 1975
Rat	Ethylmorphine N-demethylase	−	Birnbaum & Baird, 1978a,b
Rat	Ethylmorphine N-demethylase	−	Schmucker & Wang, 1980
Rat	Benzo(a)pyrene hydroxylase	−	Birnbaum & Baird, 1978a
Rat	Benzo(a)pyrene hydroxylase	=	Birnbaum & Baird, 1978b
Rat	Benzphetamine-N-demethylase	−	Birnbaum & Baird, 1978a,b
Rat	Benzphetamine-N-demethylase	−	Kao & Hudson, 1980
Rat	Epoxide hydrase	+	Birnbaum & Baird, 1979
Rat	7-Ethoxycoumarin O-deethylase	−	Kao & Hudson, 1980
Mouse	7-Ethoxycoumarin O-deethylase	−	Stohs *et al.*, 1980
Mouse	Pyroxidal kinase	=	Fonda *et al.*, 1980
Mouse	Pyridoxine-P oxidase	=	Fonda *et al.*, 1980
Mouse	Aryl hydrocarbon hydroxylase	−	Stohs *et al.*, 1980
Mouse	Aniline hydroxylase	−	Stohs *et al.*, 1980

[a] − denotes decrease with age; + denotes increase with age; = denotes no change with age.

Table VI. Changed Metabolism of Drugs with Age

Species	Drug	Change with age[a]		Reference
		in vivo	in vitro	
Rat	Carisoprodol	−	−	Kato & Takanaka, 1968c
Rat	Pentobarbital	−	−	Kato & Takanaka, 1968c
Rat	Pentobarbitone	−		Pardon et al., 1977
Mouse	Nicotine		=	Slanina & Stalhandske, 1977
Mouse	Pentobarbitone	=		Pardon et al., 1978
Mouse	Zoxazolamine		−	Baird et al., 1971

[a] − denotes decrease with age; = denotes no change with age.

old animals. Kato and Takanaka (1968c) subsequently correlated an increased duration of pentobarbital narcosis in 600-day-old Wistar rats (as compared to values in 100-day-old animals) with a decreased clearance of the barbiturate from serum and a decreased *in vitro* metabolism by liver microsomes. An increased duration of carisoprodol paralysis in the older rats was similarly correlated with a decreased clearance of this agent from the serum and brain of older male and female rats and decreased *in vitro* metabolism by liver microsomes.

These authors also found that more old than young rats convulsed and died after an acute dose of strychnine, while similar toxic signs decreased with age after OMPA (octamethylpyrophosphoramide) treatment. Both of these contrasting age effects were considered to result from decreased MFO activity since strychnine is deactivated and OMPA is activated by microsomes to an acetylcholinesterase inhibitor. In a companion paper, Kato and Takanaka (1968b) found that old rats had decreased activities of cytochrome P-450, NADPH-cytochrome P-450 reductase, NADPH oxidase, hexobarbital hydroxylase, aminopyrine N-demethylase, analine hydroxylase, strychnine oxidase and other enzymes.

Other workers using several strains of rats and mice have confirmed the above *in vivo* indicators of decreased MFO activity in old animals, i.e., barbiturate sleeping time (Baird et al., 1971, 1975, 1976; Pardon and Jones, 1978; Rolsten et al., 1979) and the increased duration of zoxazolamine paralysis (Baird et al., 1971).

Hepatic cytochrome P450, its reductase, and cytochrome b_5 are differently affected by aging. Concentrations of cytochrome P450 are either decreased (Birnbaum and Baird, 1978b; Kao and Hudson, 1980; McMartin et.al., 1980; Schmucker and Wang, 1980; Kato and Takanaka, 1968a,b) or not significantly changed by age (Baird et al., 1975; Birnbaum and Baird, 1978a; Birnbaum, 1980; Paterniti et al., 1980). Since cytochrome P450, the terminal oxidase of the MFO system, is measured as a mixture of isozymes that absorb 450 nm light after being reduced and coupled with CO, changes in one form of cytochrome P450 may mask measurement of a change in another form.

Only one out of a possible three or more forms of cytochrome P450 was shown by McMartin *et al.* (1980) to exhibit a decreased activity in microsomes from 36-month-old Wistar rats as compared to animals aged 4 and 12 months. Hepatic NADPH-cytochrome P450 reductase activity is also decreased (Kao and Hudson, 1980; Kato and Takanaka, 1968a,b; Gold and Widnell, 1974; McMartin *et al.*, 1980) or not significantly changed by aging (Birnbaum and Baird, 1978a,b; Player *et al.*, 1977). Concentrations of cytochrome b_5 were reported to be either increased (Birnbaum and Baird, 1978b; Birnbaum, 1980) or not changed (McMartin *et al.*, 1980) in old rodent livers. Other microsomal enzyme activities associated with xenobiotic metabolism and their changes with age are as follows: decreased benzphetamine N-demethylase, ethylmorphine N-demethylase and 7-ethoxycoumarin 0-demethylase and decreased or increased benzo(a)pyrene hydroxylase and zoxazolamine hydroxylase (Birnbaum and Baird, 1978a,b; Birnbaum, 1980; Baird *et al.*, 1971, 1975, 1976; Baird and Birnbaum, 1979; Kao and Hudson, 1980).

Certain chemicals such as benzo(a)pyrene and 2-fluroenamine are called procarcinogens because it is believed that it is necessary for them to be metabolized by the mixed function oxidase system to the ultimate carcinogen. Carcinogenic potential is often estimated by such short-term *in vitro* tests as covalent binding of the suspected carcinogen to DNA or induction of mutations in bacteria. Liver microsomes are often added to activate a procarcinogen to a carcinogen. In contrast to expectations one might derive from the above age changes of MFO activity, liver microsomes from older rats and mice have an increased ability to induce bacterial mutations by activating benzo(a)pyrene and 2-fluroenamine (Baird and Birnbaum, 1979) and to mediate binding of benzo(a)pyrene to DNA (Birnbaum and Baird, 1979). The increased binding of benzo(a)pyrene to DNA by microsomes from older as contrasted to younger rats occurred in spite of an unchanged level of cytochrome P450 which forms the proximate carcinogen, an increased deactivation of this carcinogen by epoxide hydrase, and unchanged glutathione-S-transferase activity in the old animals (Birnbaum and Baird, 1979).

4.4 *Biliary Excretion.* Measurements of biliary excretion depend upon a compound's uptake by the hepatocytes, its storage in the hepatocyte if uptake exceeds excretion, and its transport of the substance to the bile.

De Leeuw-Israel *et al.* (1969), and de Leeuw-Israel (1971) reported an increased bromosulfophthalein (BSP) retention in serum from 2-year-old as compared to 3-month-old female (RXU)F$_1$ rats. The increased BSP retention in the serum of old rats was ascribed to a decrease in the liver's relative storage capacity (S) for BSP, whereas the maximal excretion capacity (Tm) remained unchanged (de Leeuw-Israel, 1971). However, Kitani *et al.* (1978) observed an unchanged relative storage capacity for BSP and a decreased maximal excretion capacity in old (24 months) male Wistar rats as compared to rats aged 3 months. These discrepancies are probably due to differences in methods.

De Leeuw-Israel used the indirect method of Wheeler *et al.* (1969) to determine the S and Tm for BSP. Doubts about the reliability of this method have been expressed by McIntyre *et al.* (1973). Kitani *et al.* (1978) also reported that the maximal removal rate of indocyanine green (IcG) from serum was decreased in old Wistar rats.

In another report, Kitani *et al.* (l978a) found that the clearance of ouabain from plasma and its excretion into bile were decreased by aging in similar rats. Van Bezooijen and Knook (1978) used female WAG/Rij rats, aged 3 to 36 months, to measure *in vivo* BSP metabolism. The ability of rat liver to remove BSP from plasma decreased sharply between 3 and 12 months but remained constant thereafter. BSP storage capacity of isolated hepatocytes from these rats also decreased greatly during the first 12 months of the donor's life and slowly thereafter.

Comparison of the *in vivo* and *in vitro* data leads to the conclusion that the decrease in the liver's capacity to remove foreign substances is at least partly due to an age-related decline in storage capacity of the individual hepatocytes for those substances. Hewick *et al.* (1980) measured the biliary excretion of vitamin K_l by 90 and 477-day-old Sprague-Dawley rats having cannulated bile ducts. The excretion rate of radioactivity from labeled vitamin K_l and its metabolites was unchanged by age. Varga and Fischer (1978) found that hepatic uptake of eosin did not change significantly between 60 days and 600 days in male Sprague-Dawley rats, but that biliary excretion of this dye was maximal at 60 days, decreased one-third by 315 days and decreased a little more in the oldest (622 days) rats. Hepatic blood flow also decreased greatly up to 310 days but remained constant thereafter, ruling out decreased flow as a causative factor in later age changes in this study. Hepatic blood flow needs to be measured at more advanced ages in this and other strains of rats.

It can be concluded that compounds such as BSP, IcG and ouabain, which are not metabolized by the liver prior to biliary excretion, clearly show age-dependent changes in blood removal rates.

4.5 *Liver Blood Flow and Serum Protein Binding Capacity.* Changes in liver blood flow incurred with age are especially important for drugs or chemicals with a high extraction ratio. Examples of such drugs are chlormethiazole, labetol, lignocaine, morphine, nortryptiline, pentazocine, pethidine, propoxyphene and propanolol. Consequently, changes in blood flow with age are more significant for the age-related changes in the clearance of these drugs by the liver than changes in protein binding with age.

4.6 *Drug Uptake.* Using perfused rat liver, Kroker *et al.* (1980) observed that the hepatic uptake of bile acids was decreased to a lesser extent than their secretion in old rats. Thus, hepatic uptake is not a rate limiting step in the removal of bile acids from the blood by the liver.

4.7 *Discussion.* In studying the effect of age on the *in vivo* metabolism of drugs by the liver, many factors besides the capacity of the liver to metabolize drugs may be of importance. Even within the liver, many factors not directly related to the organelles responsible for drug metabolism play a role in the age-related changes in the capacity of the liver to metabolize drugs. Among them, changes in liver weight to body weight ratio and the spontaneous occurrence of specific liver tumors are of major importance. Studies on the excretory capacity of the liver with age indicate that compounds which are not metabolized by the liver prior to biliary excretion are removed at a slower rate by the liver with age.

Mixed function oxidase is a particularly complex biological system, because the components cytochrome P450 and NADPH-cytochrome c-reductase are multienzymatic in nature and are dependent on a continuous supply of NADPH, which is itself generated by other multienzyme systems. A serious drawback of the types of studies presented in Tables IV and V is that they were performed with microsomal preparations. In these preparations, an important part of the regulation, namely the substrate and cofactor supply, is totally absent. Diffusion of oxygen, transport of a drug or chemical to binding sites of cytochrome P450, and the delivery of NADPH to the flavoprotein may be important factors which determine the effect of age on the metabolizing capacity of the liver. As previously noted, there are indications that the metabolic processes which regulate the supply of NADPH may be unchanged with age.

Thurman and Kauffman (1980) supplied a partial list of factors that influence rates of drug metabolism in intact cells. These factors are present in the microsomes, in the cytoplasm or in the mitochondria. When using microsomal preparations, age-related changes in the cytoplasmic and mitochondrial factors will not be detected and will not influence the results. Since all of these factors are present in the *in vivo* situation, the results shown in Table VI can be indicative for age-related changes in the over-all liver drug metabolism. However, *in vivo* studies on the influence of age on the drug metabolizing capacity of the liver also have many drawbacks.

In such studies, complicating extrahepatic factors such as neurological, endocrinological, and circulatory disturbances may influence the metabolic capacity of the liver with age. In addition, changes in drug absorption, drug distribution and kidney function with age should be taken into account when reaching conclusions about age-related changes in the liver metabolic capacity in rodents.

In view of the limitations for the *in vivo* studies mentioned above, an experimental system based on the use of isolated intact hepatocytes has the advantage that extrahepatic influences can be excluded and that they contain all cellular factors involved in drug metabolism. Many recent articles indicate (for reviews, see Billings *et al.*, 1977; Anderson *et al.*, 1978; Thurman and Kauffman, 1980; and Sirica and Pitot, 1980) that metabolism of compounds by hepatocytes isolated from young rats clearly resembles *in vivo* metabolic rates. In addition, age-related changes in interactions between intermediate metabolism and mixed function oxidation can be investigated by using hepatocytes isolated from rats or mice of different ages. Therefore, data obtained on the drug metabolic capacity of those isolated hepatocytes can be expected to provide useful information on the role of the liver in age-related changes of drug metabolism kinetics of rodents *in vivo*. Such studies have not been performed up to now. The metabolism of digitoxin by isolated hepatocytes recently has been investigated (van Bezooijen *et al.*, 1980). Preliminary data on the capacity of hepatocytes isolated from rats of different ages reveal no qualitative changes in the pattern of digitoxin metabolites with age.

5. Renal Excretion

Many chemicals are eliminated from the body into the urine via filtration through glomeruli or secretion into tubules of the kidney. The physiological measurements of glomerular filtration rate (GFR) and p-aminohippuric (PAH) transport can be used to indicate the efficacy of xenobiotic elimination by the kidney.

The effects of aging on renal function are complicated by the glomerulonephrosis that arises spontaneously in certain strains of rats. This may account for the discrepancy in reports on the effect of aging on GFR. Alt *et al.* (1980) found that GFR decreased 70% between the ages of 6 and 38 months in male Han:Wistar rats. Their older rats also exhibited proteinuria and histologically verified severe glomerulonephrosis. In contrast, Bengele *et al.* (1981) state that GFR was not changed by aging from 4 to 23 months in male F344 rats even though urine concentrating ability was diminished in the older animals. GFR was also unchanged in female Wistar rats aged 12, 24 and 30 months (Gregory and Barrows, 1969). Tubular excretion of PAH *in vivo* was decreased by aging in these rats. The *in vitro* maximal accumulation of PAH, but not its rate of uptake, was progressively decreased in kidney slices from old (28 months) and middle-aged (14 months) as compared to young (3 months) female Sprague-Dawley rats (Adams and Barrows, 1963). *In vitro* accumulation of PAH into kidney slices from male Wistar rats was also found by Tucker *et al.* (1976) to be decreased as the age of the donor increased from 12 to 24 months. Restriction of dietary protein prevented this decrease.

VI. Duration of Long-Term Studies

In recent years, there has been some consideration given to extending chronic toxicity/cancer studies beyond the traditional 24 months for rats and 18 months for mice. The need or desirability for extending studies beyond these periods is questionable. Several factors should be taken into account in reviewing this issue, including the changing health status in aging animals, the induction time for chemically induced tumors, the time of occurrence of toxic effects other than carcinogenicity, and the cost of extending toxicity studies. The latter is considered in detail in Section VII of this monograph. The other factors to be considered in extending toxicity studies are discussed below.

A very compelling reason for not extending studies beyond 24 months is the need to adhere to a very important basic principle and requirement in toxicity testing, namely the use of healthy animals. Particular attention is paid to the use of healthy animals in most phases of the conduct of toxicity studies. Every precaution is taken to obtain healthy animals from a reliable source. The animals are shipped under prescribed conditions that minimize the likelihood of developing disease during this period. They are examined for a host of disease entities prior to being placed on test and are maintained under conditions that are ideal for maintaining a healthy status. The sole objective of all these considerable efforts is to provide a healthy animal for toxicity testing. In this regard, it is as important to use a pure biological system (the healthy animal) as it is to use chemicals of known composition and purity. Since various diseases might alter the toxicity of a chemical in various ways, the "true" toxicity of the chemical may not be appreciated unless the test is done in a healthy animal. It is important that this principle be applied to all age groups.

Many of the common diseases of rodents that are associated with aging alter the function of several organs or systems as well as the specific target organ. For example, in chronic progressive nephropathy, a very common disease of rats, secondary lesions are observed in the liver, parathyroid, lungs, heart, blood vessels, and gastro-intestinal tract. Many clinical chemistry values for blood are secondarily altered because of the primary disease or its sequelae. The more the animal is thus affected, the less likely it would serve as a useful biological model. In addition, there is a good possibility that subtle chronic effects might be "masked" or "hidden" if they occurred in an organ that was markedly altered by a common aging disease. If during the course of investigations it becomes important to know how a particular chemical might be handled by humans with certain aging disease entities, then a suitable animal model for the human disease condition should be sought. This requires a special study quite distinct from the standard chronic toxicity or carcinogenicity studies.

Studies over the past few years, that have been conducted for more than 24 months, indicate that for a number of common spontaneous tumors, the incidence increased markedly with increasing age. When the incidence in control animals is very high, the study is exceedingly difficult to assess properly.

As the health of aging animals slowly but progressively deteriorates, it becomes increasingly difficult to determine when an animal is likely to die. The likelihood of losing animals due to autolysis because of unanticipated death becomes more likely the longer the animals are maintained on test.

Guidelines basing extension on the number of animals living at certain time periods after 24 months do not take into account the cause of death of the animals. As outlined above, disease process can profoundly alter homeostasis and consequently alter the animal's ability to deal with toxic chemicals. The value of data derived from such animals is of very questionable value for safety assessment purposes.

Another reason for extending studies beyond 24 months would be that evidence of carcinogenicity might be seen only after 24 months. The authors of this monograph are not aware of any examples where the maximum tolerated dose of a chemical was included in a dosing regimen to either mice, rats or hamsters in an adequate carcinogenicity or chronic toxicity study and in which evidence of carcinogenicity was not apparent or suspect prior to 24 months. To obtain definitive data in this regard the IARC monographs Volume 1 to Volume 29 (excluding Volume 28) were reviewed.

IARC monograph supplement 1 (1979) lists 142 chemicals reviewed in Volumes 1 to 20 for which there was sufficient evidence for carcinogenicity. When the data from Volumes 21 to 29 are included with the first 20 volumes there are 179 chemicals for which sufficient evidence for carcinogenicity exists. The data on these 179 chemicals were reviewed to determine when evidence of carcinogenicity was first observed. In some instances the time of appearance of the first relevant tumors was given in the monographs. In other instances it was reported that a certain percentage of animals had developed the relevant tumors by a specified time period. In the latter instance the first tumors would be seen prior to the specified time period, nevertheless for the purpose of this review the specified time period was taken as the time when there was first evidence of carcinogenicity. From this information the time at which relevant tumors were first observed was designated as prior to 6, 12, 18, or 24 months. The results are given in the following table:

Time in months at which evidence of tumors was first observed

	6	12	18	24
No. of Chemicals	72	153	171	179
Percent	40.2	85.4	95.4	100

From the table it may be seen that for over 85% of the chemicals there was evidence of carcinogenicity prior to 12 months and for over 95% of the chemicals there was evidence prior to 18 months. There was evidence for carcinogenicity before 24 months in all instances. It should be noted that in many of the studies reported, interim kills were not included in the study design so that it is reasonable to suggest that the latency period for tumors was likely shorter than indicated in the table. Furthermore for those tumors with associated preneoplastic change, evidence of a carcinogenic potential would be present prior to the time periods listed in the table. Even the so-called weak carcinogens such as saccharin provide evidence of carcinogenicity before 24 months. In the study by Arnold *et al.* (1980) the first bladder tumors in the F_1 generation were observed at 17 months and 21 months in the F_0 generation.

It would appear that the traditional 18 months for mice and 24 months for rats is an adequate duration for carcinogenicity studies. However, protocols should be flexible to the extent that if evidence of carcinogenicity appears late in the study, the study could be extended for a few additional months with a view to obtaining statistically significant results.

VII. Cost of Conducting Toxicity Studies with Durations of 18, 24 or 30 Months

1. Calculating the Cost of Long-Term Studies

The cost of conducting long-term studies is based on the total workload in the study and on the duration of the study. In order to determine the cost of 18, 24 or 30-month studies, a number of laboratories were polled including industry, private contract and government laboratories.

1.1 *How Costs Were Calculated.* It is difficult to provide exact costs that compare one laboratory to another because of the variation in overhead, time accounting, number of personnel involved, etc. Nevertheless, it is possible to provide a rough comparison of the change in cost of an 18, 24 or 30-month study, at least in relative terms. Before calculating the cost of such studies in different laboratories, several assumptions were made which are listed below.

1. Uniform survival of the animals placed on test at six weeks of age is expected.
2. Animals are housed two per cage and isolated in an animal room during the entire conduct of the study.
3. Cleaning is performed every two days and animals are transferred to clean cages on a monthly basis.
4. Water is provided by an automatic watering system, and food by *ad libitum*.
5. Fifty rats/sex/dose are used with three dose levels, plus a control.
6. At least one interim kill will take place which utilizes a minimum of five animals/sex/dose level.
7. Body weights and food consumption data from a representative group of animals are determined weekly, and these data are used to adjust the concentration of test diets weekly to maintain dosages of a mg/kg to body weight on a daily basis.

8. The calculations are for a diet study (i.e. not an inhalation study).
9. Body weights and food consumption data are recorded weekly during the first three months of the study and monthly thereafter.
10. Test diets are mixed every two weeks and analysis of the test diets are performed quarterly during the duration of the study.
11. The test material is analyzed quarterly to confirm the composition.
12. Observation of the animals and the cages in rooms involved are observed twice daily.
13. Animals are palpated for masses once per month beginning on the sixth month of the study.
14. Good laboratory practices are followed and quality assurance audits are performed quarterly during the conduct of the study.
15. All animals dying spontaneously are submitted for gross pathological examination and subsequent histopathologic examination.
16. The cost of necropsy and histopathology examination for scheduled sacrifices are considered proportional to the percent mortality, since increased spontaneous lesions are proportional to the mortality.

1.2 *Why the Costs Increase with Age of Animals.* As animals become older the cost per animal becomes greater. Some of the factors that lead to increased cost and increased complications during long-term studies are listed below.

1. When increased palpable masses occur during a study, more time is required to examine the animals and to tabulate the increased data for the in-life portion of the study.
2. Older animals will develop other clinical effects such as perineal soiling, soiling around the eyes, rough hair coats, etc. All of these lesions continue to compound themselves during the study and also need to be recorded and evaluated during the conduct of a study.
3. There is a need for more frequent observations as the animals become older. When that point in the survival curve where mortality increases is reached, a minimum of two examinations is often needed per day, seven days a week, in order to cull moribund animals to prevent or reduce autolysis and cannibalization. This means that as the animals are on test for increasingly longer periods of time, there is an increasing requirement for the services of highly trained personnel.
4. Although fewer animals are on test, they still utilize the same amount of space during the long-term study. The older animals tie up a disproportionate number of cages, racks, animal rooms and personnel. While the older population of animals represents fewer animals on test, overhead for utilization of rooms, cages, etc. remains the same.
5. When animal rooms are tied up for longer periods of time in order to complete a single study, the utilization of resources is disproportionately

greater, which reduces the number of long-term studies that can be initiated and new compounds that can be evaluated.

6. More lesions and diseases occur in older animals, which markedly increases the cost of the pathologic examination involved. It takes more time to do a gross examination on an older animal than it does a young animal. This ties up several people in the necropsy room including the pathologist, who then spend less time on the evaluation of other studies. Not only does it take more time to perform the gross examination on old versus young animals, but more time is also required to trim the tissues, and more blocks and slides are needed because there are more lesions to examine. It takes more time to evaluate the histopathology slides and, as a result, much more time is needed to tabulate, interpret and report the data from the studies on the older versus the younger animals.

7. More lesions in the older animals increase the difficulty in determining a compound-related effect versus an effect due to biological variability (i.e. natural variations in spontaneously occurring lesions).

2. Results of the Survey

The results of the survey involving six laboratories indicated considerable variability from laboratory to laboratory because of the variable factors outlined in the preceding paragraphs. Despite this, the actual cost estimates were very close.

Duration of Study in Months	Per Animal Cost in 1981 Dollars Average Cost (Range) from Six Laboratories
18	$ 735.00 (700 to 859)
24	$ 908.00 (795 to 1100)
30	$1131.00 (895 to 1500)

As can be seen from the above data, the longer the studies are conducted, the greater the cost per unit animal. If 500 animals are studied, then the cost at 18 months is approximately $370,000 compared to $570,000 at 30 months. As the long-term studies are evaluated, it is clear that we must not only look at the data obtained from the studies but also, at some point, examine the costs to conduct the studies and whether the cost to conduct longer and longer studies exceeds the value of reliable and reproducible data that can be obtained. In addition to the increased costs, the increased age of animals leads to an increase in geriatric diseases which affect their utility as acceptable experimental models. The prevalence of geriatric diseases greatly complicates assessment of any changes that may be induced by a test compound.

VIII. Conclusions

Traditionally, long-term rat studies have been of 24 months duration and long-term mouse studies have been of 18 to 24 months duration. There has been a growing trend to routinely extend long-term studies beyond 24 months or to terminate when a defined percent mortality has occurred in one or more groups of animals. It is clear that by extending these studies, any data that is obtained is complicated by the expected or normal geriatric changes which occur in the animal population. Since geriatric changes are often species specific and can alter the metabolic capabilities of the test animal, then meaningful extrapolation of the findings to other species is questionable. The longer the studies are conducted, the more design problems, the greater the cost, and the greater the inability to separate induced changes from spontaneous background changes.

Studies in aged rodents with geriatric diseases may have little or no relevance to humans because most geriatric diseases of the aged rodent are different from those of the aged human. There are few diseases in old rats and mice that have suitable human counterparts. Currently there is a lack of scientific evidence to support extending studies beyond the traditional 24 month period. Studies terminated by 24 months are evaluating animals that are relatively healthy and are just beginning to enter the stage where geriatric diseases are increasing.

Because rats and mice can live to 3 or more years, studies terminated at 24 months do not examine the effects in truly aged animals. To do this properly would require testing rodents that did not succumb to a disease of old age until they were 3 years of age or older. Conducting such studies would be prohibitively expensive since the commonly used strains all have a high background of diseases that are peculiar to the strain. These diseases occur at varying incidences so that in order to obtain a sufficient number of animals free of disease at 3 years would require initiating the studies with very large numbers of animals. For example, the F344 rat has a high background of spontaneously occurring leukemia. At 24 months the incidence may be approximately 20%, but by 30 months it can be as high as 50%. Therefore, half of the animals have only minimal value. To compensate for this loss, more rats would have to be added at the start of the study to assure survival of a meaningful number of rats free of leukemia at the end of a 30 month study.

The issue of testing compounds in geriatric animals is important. However, due to the marked species variations in the spontaneous geriatric diseases, it is extremely difficult to find a suitable animal model that truly represents the aged human. The issue of studying compounds in geriatric animal populations should not be ignored. Rather, new protocols and experimental approaches are needed to evaluate changes in drug toxicity, metabolism and pharmacokinetics in young versus geriatric populations of humans or animals. But, this is not the purpose of the traditional chronic toxicity or oncogenicity studies. The traditional chronic toxicity and carcinogenicity bioassay was not designed to study effects in geriatric populations. Since it is standard practice to conduct toxicity studies on healthy animals, long-term toxicity studies should be no exception. Long-term studies should be conducted in animals before the background geriatric diseases increase to a point where such diseases make any data interpretation unsound and meaningless.

IX. Areas in Need of Future Research

A number of studies are needed in order to compare and to evaluate young versus old populations of animals and how drugs or chemicals are handled. Such information is needed in order to make an adequate safety evaluation of the compound in question. These studies include the following:

1. Studies to correlate morphological organ changes with functional and biochemical alterations with age.
2. Studies to compare drug or chemical metabolism in young, middle-aged and old rodents.
3. Studies to compare acute and subchronic toxicity of young and old test animals.
4. Studies to determine if old animals have longer or shorter latency periods for cancer when given known carcinogens.
5. Studies to compare multi-organ effects produced by a disease process or toxic change in a primary target tissue or organ.
6. Studies to determine the most appropriate age of animals that provide a reasonable safety assessment for chronic effects in older humans.
7. Studies to determine how to evaluate the safety of chemicals for the geriatric human population.
8. Cell culture studies to help determine if cells from old and young animals handle drugs in the same way.

X. Summary

Because of improved selection and animal husbandry, rodents used in long-term toxicity studies live longer than those used in studies in past decades. The 50% survival rate of most rodents is about 27-30 months of age, so that the traditional 24-month study (animals are 25 to 26 months old) approaches this 50% survival figure.

A variety of age-associated diseases are commonly encountered in laboratory animals used for chronic toxicity testing. With increasing age of the animal, diseases increase in severity and incidence, so that homeostasis may eventually become markedly altered.

The disease processes are associated with alterations in organ function and morphology making it difficult to distinguish between natural disease and chemically induced toxicity. Under these circumstances, the evaluation of the toxic effects of test chemicals becomes difficult, and attempts at realistic extrapolation of the findings to humans are seriously compromised.

Geriatric changes in organ function and morphology are associated with changes in metabolism, and this, in turn, can alter the response to chemical toxicities. Although there are exceptions, in general the aging animal metabolizes chemicals less effectively and is more susceptible to toxic effects of chemicals. Changes in absorption, plasma concentration, tissue binding and excretion may occur with advancing years. These changes and their assessment are complicated by disease processes.

Because the liver is responsible quantitatively and qualitatively for the metabolism of more xenobiotics than any other organ, geriatric changes in the liver are of particular interest. Changes in liver weight with increasing age result in changes in the capacity of the liver to metabolize chemicals. The increase in ploidy of the liver cell nucleus, that is seen with increasing age in rodents, could result in a decrease in the amount of cell surface per unit volume. This, in turn, may decrease the rate of chemical uptake by the liver.

Results in studies in rats on changes involving various hepatic enzymes suggest that alterations in activity may occur with advancing age.

Biliary excretion changes with age. There is a decrease in the liver's capacity to remove foreign substance in older animals, and this may be due in part to an age-related decline in the storage capacity of the individual hepatocytes.

Hepatic blood flow decreases with age, and this is associated with changes in clearances of chemicals, particularly those with a high extraction ratio.

Aging, toxicity, and carcinogenicity are complex biological processes. An alteration in any one can lead to changes in another. Some parameters may be increased while others are decreased. Exposure can cause a shift in these complex biological processes.

Although there has been a trend towards increasing the duration of studies, in light of existing scientific evidence, there is little data to support extending studies for longer than the traditional 24 months. Studies beyond 18 months in mice and 24 months in rats result in greater variability in the studies, less reliability and greater difficulty in interpretation of the data obtained, and less likelihood that studies can be reproduced.

XI. References

Abel, E.L. (1978). Effects of ethanol and pentobarbital in mice of different ages. *Physiol. Psychol.* 6, 366-368.

Adams, J.R. and Barrows, C.H. (1963). Effect of age on PAH accumulation by kidney slices of female rats. *J. Gerontol.* 18, 37-40.

Adelman, R.C. (1971). Age-dependent effects in enzyme induction - a biochemical expression of aging. *Exp. Gerontol.* 6, 75-87.

Ali, M., Nicholls, P.J., and Yoosuf, A. (1979). The influence of old age and of renal failure on hepatic glucuronidation in the rat. *Brit. J. Pharmacol.* 66, 498-499.

Alt, J.M., Hackbarth, H., Deerberg, F. and Stolte, H. (1980). Proteinuria in rats in relation to age-dependent renal changes. *Lab. Anim.* 14, 95-101.

Altman, N.H. and Goodman, D. (1979). Neoplastic diseases of the laboratory rat. In *The Laboratory Rat: Volume I, Biology and Diseases* (H.J. Baker, J.R. Lindsey and S. Weisbroth, eds.) pp. 333-376, Academic Press, New York.

Anderson, B., Berggren, M. and Moldeus, P. (1978). Conjugation of various drugs in isolated hepatocytes. *Drug Metab. Dispos.* 6, 611-616.

Andrew, W. and Pruett, D. (1957). Senile changes in the kidneys of Wistar Institute rats. *Am. J. Anat.* 100, 51.

Anver, M.R. and Cohen, B.J. (1979). Lesions associated with aging. In *The Laboratory Rat: Volume I, Biology and Diseases* (H.J. Baker, J.R. Lindsey and S.H. Weisbroth, eds.) pp. 378-399, Academic Press. New York.

Aoki, T., Teller, M.N. and Robitallie, M.L. (1965). Aging and carcinogenesis. II. Effect of age on phagocytic activity of the reticuloendothelial system and on tumor growth. *J. Nat. Cancer Inst.* 34, 255-264.

Arakaw, M. (1970). A scanning electron microscopy of the glomerulus of normal and nephrotic rats. *Lab. Invest.* 23, 489-496.

Arakaw, M. and Tokunaga, J. (1972). A scanning electron microscope study of the glomerulus. Further consideration of the mechanism of the fusion of podocyte terminal processes in nephrotic rats. *Lab. Invest.* 27, 366-371.

Arnold, D.L., Charbonneau, S.M., Zawidzka, Z.Z. and Grice, H.C. (1977). Monitoring animal health during chronic toxicity studies. *J. Eviron. Pathol. Toxicol.* 1, 227-239.

Arnold, D.L., Moodie, C.A., Grice, H.C., Charbonneau, S.M., Stavric, B., Collins, B.T., McGuire, P.F. Zawidzka, Z.Z. and Munro, I.C. (1980). Long- term toxicity of ortho-toluenesulfonamide and sodium saccharin in the rat. *Toxicol. Appl. Pharmcol.* 52, 113-152.

Baird, M.B. and Birnbaum, L.S. (1979). Increased production of mutagenic metabolites of carcinogens by tissues from senescent rodents. *Cancer Res.* 39, 4752-4755.

Baird, M.B., Nicolosi, R.J., Massie, H.R. and Samis, H.V. (1975). Microsomal mixed-function oxidase activity and senescence - I. Hexobarbital sleep time and induction of components of the hepatic microsomal enzyme system in rats of different ages. *Exp. Gerontol.* 10, 89-99.

Baird, M.B., Samis, H.V. and Massie, H.R.(1971). Recovery from zoxazolamine paralysis and metabolism *in vitro* of zoxazolamine in aging mice. *Nature* 233, 565-566.

Baird, M.B., Zimmerman, J.A., Massie, H.R. and Pacilio, L.V. (1976). Microsomal mixed function oxidase activity and senescence - II. *In vivo* and *in vitro* hepatic drug metabolism in rats of different ages following partial hepatectomy. *Exp. Gerontol.* 11, 161-165.

Bengele, H.H., Mathias, R.S., Perkins, J.H. and Alexander, E.A. (1981). Urinary concentrating defect in the aged rat. *Amer. J. Physiol.* 240, F147-F150.

Berg, B.N. (1967). Longevity studies in rats. II. Pathology of aging rats. In *Pathology of Laboratory Rats and Mice* (E. Cotchin and F.J.C. Roe, eds.) Chapter 23, pp. 749-786, Blackwell Scientific Publications, Oxford and Edinburgh.

Berg, B.N. and Simms, H.S. (1960). Nutrition and longevity in the rat. II. Longevity and onset of disease with different levels of food intake. *J. Nutr.* 71, 255-263.

Berg, B.N. and Simms, H.S. (1961). Nutrition and longevity in the rat. III. Food restriction beyond 800 days. *J. Nutr.* 74, 23-32.

Berg, B.N. and Simms, H.S. (1965). Nutrition, onset of disease, and longevity in the rat. *Can. Med. Assoc. J.* 93, 911-913.

Bilder, G.E. (1975). Studies on immune competence in the rat: changes with age, sex and strain. *J. Gerontol.* 30, 641-646.

Billings, R.E., McMahon, R.E., Ashmore, J. and Wagle, S.R. (1977). The metabolism of drugs in isolated rat hepatocytes. *Drug Metab. Dispos.* 5, 518-526.

Birnbaum, L.S. (1980). Altered hepatic drug metabolism in senescent mice. *Exp. Gerontol.* 15, 259-267.

Birnbaum, L.S. and Baird, M.B. (1978a). Induction of hepatic mixed function oxidases in senescent rodents - II. Effect of polychlorinated biphenyls. *Exp. Gerontol.* 13, 469-477.

Birnbaum, L.S. and Baird, M.B. (1978b). Induction of hepatic mixed function oxidases in senescent rodents. *Exp. Gerontol.* 13, 299-303.

Birnbaum, L.S. and Baird, M.B. (1979). Senescent changes in rodent hepatic epoxide metabolism. *Chem. Biol. Interact.* 26, 245-256.

Blankwater, M.J. (1978). Ageing and the humoral immune response in mice. Ph.D. Thesis, University of Utrecht, The Netherlands.

Bolten, W.K., Benton, F.R., Maclay, J.G. and Sturgill, B.C. (1976). Spontaneous glomerular sclerosis in aging Sprague-Dawley rats. *Am. J. Pathol.* 85, 277-300.

Boorman, G.A. and Hollander, C.F. (1972). Occurrence of spontaneous cancer with aging in an inbred strain of rats. *TNO Nieuws* 27, 692-695.

Boorman, G.A. and Hollander, C.F. (1973). Spontaneous lesions in the female WAG/Rij (Wistar) rat. *J. Gerontol.* 28, 152-159.

Brouwer, A. and Knook, D.L. (1983). The reticuloendothelial system: a review. Accepted for publication *Mech. Ageing Dev.* 15.

Bullock, B.C., Banks, K.L. and Manning, P.J. (1968). Common lesions in the aged rat. In *The Laboratory Animal in Gerontological Research* (T.W. Harris, ed.) Publ. No. 1591, pp. 62-82, National Academy of Sciences, Washington.

Burek, J.D. (1978). *Pathology of Aging Rats: A Morphological and Experimental Study of the Age-Associated Lesions in Aging BN/Bi, WAG/Rij and (WAG x BN)F₁ Rats.* CRC Press, Inc., West Palm Beach.

Burek, J.D. and Hollander, C.F. (1977). Incidence patterns of spontaneous tumors in BN/Bi rats. *J. Nat. Cancer Inst.* 58, 99-105.

Burek, J.D. and Hollander, C.F. (1980). Experimental gerontology. In *The Laboratory Rat: Volume II, Research Applications* (H.J. Baker, J.R. Lindsay and S. Weisbroth, eds.) pp. 149-159, Academic Press, New York.

Burek, J.D., Molello, J.A. and Warner, S.D. (1982). Selected nonneoplastic diseases. In *The Mouse in Biomedical Research* (H.L. Foster, J.D. Small and J.G. Fox, eds.) Vol. II, Chapter 23, pp. 425-440, Academic Press, New York.

Burek, J.D., Quast, J.F., Dittenber, D.A. and Bell, T.J. (1979). Structural functional correlations in chronic renal failure in the rat. Symposium, "Renal Disease" American College of Veterinary Pathologists, Denver.

Burek, J.D., van der Kogel, A.J. and Hollander, C.F. (1976). Degenerative myelopathy in three strains of aging rats. *Vet. Pathol.* 13, 321-331.

Calingaert, A. and Zorzoli, A. (1965). The influence of age on 6-deoxy-D-glucose accumulation by mouse intestine. *J. Gerontol.* 20, 211-214.

Cohen, B.J. and Anver, M.R. (1976). Pathological changes during aging in the rat. In *Special Review of Experimental Aging Research: Progress in Biology* (M.F. Elias, B.E. Eleftheriou, and P.K. Elias, eds.), pp. 379-403, Beech Hill, Mt. Desert.

Coleman, G.L., Barthold, S.W., Osbaldiston, G.W., Foster, S.J. and Jonas, A.M. (1977). Pathological changes during aging in barrier-reared Fischer 344 male rats. *J. Gerontol.* 32, 258-278.

Coniglio, J.J., Liu, D.S.H. and Richardson, A. (1979). A comparison of protein synthesis by liver parenchymal cells isolated from Fischer F344 rats of various ages. *Mech. Ageing Dev.* 11, 77-90.

Conway, P., Valentovic, M. and Bachmann, K. (1979). Tissue binding of warfarin. *Res. Commun. Chem. Pathol. Pharmacol.* 26, 309-315.

Cotchin, E. and Roe, F.J.C. (1967). *Pathology of Laboratory Rats and Mice,* Blackwell Scientific Publications, Oxford and Edinburgh.

Couser, W.G. and Stilmant, M.M. (1975). Mesangial lesions and focal glomerular sclerosis in the aging rat. *Lab. Invest.* 33, 491-501.

Couser, W.B. and Stilmant, M.M. (1976). The immunopathology of the aging rat kidney. *J. Gerontol.* 31, 13-22.

Crain, R.C. (1958). Spontaneous tumors in the Rochester strain of Wistar rat. *Am. J. Pathol.* 34, 311-335.

de Leeuw-Israel, F.R. (1971). Aging Changes in the Rat Liver. An Experimental Study of Hepatocellular Function and Morphology, Ph.D. Thesis, University of Leiden, The Netherlands.

de Leeuw-Israel, F.R., Hollander, C.F. and Arp-Neefjes, J.M. (1969). Hepatic storage and maximal biliary excretion of bromosulphalein (BSP) in young and old rats. *J. Gerontol.* 24, 140-142.

Den Engelse, L., Hollander, C.F. and Misdorp, W. (1974). A sex-dependent difference in the type of tumours induced by dimethylnitrosamine in the livers of C3Hf mice. *Europ. J. Cancer* 10, 129-135.

Deringer, M.K. (1956). The effect of subcutaneous inoculation of 4-o-tolylazo-o-toloidine in strain HR mice. *J. Nat. Cancer Inst.* 17, 533-539.

Elema, J.D. and Arends, A. (1975). Focal and segmental glomerular hyalinosis and sclerosis in the rat. *Lab. Invest.* 33, 554-561.

Epstein, M. (1979). Effects of aging on the kidney. *Fed. Proc.* 38, 168-172.

Finch, C.E. (1976). The regulation of physiological changes during mammalian aging. *Q. Rev. Biol.* 51, 49-83.

Finch, C.E. (1979) Neuroendocrine mechanisms and aging. *Fed. Proc.* 38, 178-183.

Fonda, M.L., Eggers, D.K. and Mehta, R. (1980). Vitamin B-6 metabolism in the livers of young adult and senescent mice. *Exp. Gerontol.* 15, 457-463.

Fox, J.G. (1977). Clinical assessment of laboratory rodents on long-term bioassay studies. *J. Environ. Path. Toxicol.* 1, 199-226.

Gellatly, J.B.M. (1967). Discussion in *Pathology of Laboratory Rats and Mice* (E. Cotchin and F.J.C. Roe, eds.), p. 22. Blackwell Scientific Publications, Oxford and Edinburgh.

Gilbert, C. and Gillman, J. (1958). Spontaneous neoplasms in the albino rat. *S. Afr. J. Med. Sci.* 23, 257-272.

Gillette, J.R. (1979). Biotransformation of drugs during aging. *Fed. Proc.* 38, 1900-1909.

Gold, G. and Widnell, C.C. (1974). Reversal of age-related changes in microsomal enzyme activities following the administration of triamcinolone, triiodothyronine and phenobarbital. *Biochem. Biophys. Acta.* 334, 75-85.

Gray, J.E. (1977). *Chronic Progressive Nephrosis in the Albino Rat.* CRC Critical Reviews in Toxicology, pp. 115-144, CRC Press, Inc., West Palm Beach.

Gray, J.E., van Zwieten, M.J. and Hollander, C.F. (1982). Early light microscopic changes of chronic progressive nephrosis in several strains of aging laboratory rats. *J. Gerontol.* 37, 142-150.

Gray, J.E., Weaver, R.N., and Purmalis, A. (1974). Ultrastructural observations of chronic progressive nephrosis in the Sprague-Dawley rat. *Vet. Pathol.* 11, 153-164.

Greenberg, L.H. and Weiss, B. (1979). Ability of aged rats to alter *beta* adrenergic receptors of brain in response to repeated administration of reserpine and desmethylimipramine. *J. Pharm. Exp. Therap.* 211, 309-316.

Gregory, J.G. and Barrows, C.H. (1969). The effect of age on renal functions of female rats. *J. Gerontol.* 24, 321-323.

Grinna, L.S. and Barber, A.A. (1972). Age-related changes in membrane lipid content and enzyme activities. *Biochim. Biophys. Acta.* 288, 347-353.

Gsell, D. (1964). Absterbekurven und Wachstumscharakteristika einer "Alterszucht" von Wistar-Ratten. *Int. Z. Vitaminforsch.* 9, 114-125.

Hess, R., Keberle, H., Koella, W.P., Schmid, K.and Gelzer, J. (1972). Clioquinol: absence of neurotoxicity in laboratory animals. *Lancet, II,* 424-425.

Hewick, D.S., Shepherd, A.M.M., Stevenson, I.H. and Wilson, N.M. (1980). Pharmacokinetics of vitamin K in young and aged rats. *Brit. J. Pharmacol.* 69, 310P-311P.

Hirokawa, H. (1975). Characterization of age-associated kidney disease in Wistar rats. *Mech. Ageing Dev.* 4, 301-316.

Hollander, C.F. (1970). Functional and cellular aspects of organ ageing. *Exp. Gerontol.* 5, 313-321.

Hollander, D. and Morgan, D. (1979). Aging: its influence on vitamin A intestinal absorption *in vivo* by the rat. *Exp. Gerontol.* 14, 301-305.

Hoover, K.L., Ward, J.M. and Stinson, S.F. (1980). Histopathologic differences between liver tumors in untreated (C57Bl/6 x C3H)F$_1$ (B6C3F$_1$) mice and nitrogen-fed mice. *J. Nat. Cancer Inst.* 65, 937-948.

Horita, N., Ishii, T. and Izumiyama, Y. (1980). Ultrastructure of 6-aminonicotinamide (6-AN)-induced lesions in the central nervous system of rats. *Acta.Neuropathol.* (Berl.) 49, 19-27.

Itakura, C., Iida, M. and Goto, M. (1977). Renal secondary hyperparathyroidism in aged Sprague-Dawley rats. *Vet. Pathol.* 14, 463-469.

Jacobs, B.B. and Dieter, D.K. (1978). Spontaneous hepatomas in mice inbred from Ha:ICR Swiss stock: effects of sex, cedar shaving in bedding, and immunization with fetal liver or hepatoma cells. J. *Nat. Cancer Inst.* 61, 1531-1534.

Jacobs, B.B. and Huseby, R.A. (1967). Neoplasms occurring in aged Fischer rats with special reference to testicular, uterine and thyroid tumors. *J. Nat. Cancer Inst.* 39, 303-309.

Jaroslow, B.N. and Larrick, J.W. (1973). Clearance of foreign red cells from the blood of aging mice. *Mech. Ageing Dev.* 2, 23-32.

Jones, E.L., Searle, C.E. and Smith, W.T. (1973). Peripheral neuropathy in ageing rats fed clioquinol and a maize diet. *Acta.Neuropath. (Berl.)* 24, 256-262.

Jones, T.C. (1967). Pathology of the liver of rats and mice. In *Pathology of Laboratory Rats and Mice* (E. Cotchin and F.J.C. Roe, eds.) pp. 1-23, Blackwell Scientific Publications, Oxford and Edinburgh.

Jones, T.C. (1967b). Pathology of the liver of rats and mice. Discussion of J.B.M. Gellatly. In *Pathology of Laboratory Rats and Mice* (E. Cotchin and F.J.C. Roe, eds.) pp. 22, Blackwell Scientific Publications, Oxford and Edinburgh.

Jones, T.W.G. and Pardon, I.S. (1980). The effect of age on the plasma protein binding of pentobarbitone in the mouse. A brief note. *Mech. Ageing Dev.* 14, 409-415.

Kao, J. and Hudson, P. (1980). Induction of the hepatic cytochrome P450-dependent mono-oxygenase system in young and geriatric rats. *Biochem. Pharmacol.* 29, 1191-1194.

Kato, R. and Takanaka, A. (1968a). Effect of phenobarbital on electron transport system, oxidation and reduction of drugs in liver microsomes of rats of different ages. *J. Biochem.* 63, 406-408.

Kato, R. and Takanaka, A. (1968b). Metabolism of drugs in old rats (I). Activities of NADPH-linked electron transport and drug-metabolizine enzyme systems in liver microsomes of old rats. *Jap. J. Pharmacol.* 18, 381-388.

Kato, R. and Takanaka, A. (1968c). Metabolism of drugs in old rats (II). Metabolism *in vivo* and effect of drugs in old rats. *Jap. J. Pharmacol.* 18, 389-396.

Kitani, K. (1977). Functional aspects of the ageing liver. In *Liver and Ageing* (D. Platt ed.) pp. 5-17, F.K. Schattauer Verlag, Stuttgart and New York.

Kitani, K., Kanai, S. and Miura, R. (1978). Hepatic metabolism of sulfobromophthalein (BSP) and indocyanine green (IcG) in aging rats. In *Liver and Aging* (K. Kitani, ed.) pp. 145-156, Elsevier/North-Holland Biomedical Press, Amsterdam, New York, Oxford.

Kitani, K., Kanai, S., Miura, R., Morita, Y. and Kasahara, M. (1978a). The effect of aging on the biliary excretion of ouabain in the rat. *Exp. Gerontol.* 13, 9-17.

Kitani, K., Zurcher, C., and van Bezooijen, C.F.A. (1982). The effect of aging on the hepatic metabolism of sufobromophthalein in BN/Bi female and WAG/Rij male and female rats. *Mech. Ageing Dev.* 7, 381-393.

Klimas, J.E. (1968). Intestinal glucose absorption during the life-span of a colony of rats. *J. Gerontol.* 23, 529-532.

Klotz, U. (1979). Effect of age on levels of diazepam in plasma and brain of rats. *Naunyn-Schmiedeberg's Arch.* 307, 167-169.

Knook, D.L. and Sleyster, E.Ch. (1976). Lysosomal enzyme activities in parenchymal and non-parenchymal liver cells isolated from young, adult and old rats. *Mech. Ageing Dev.* 5, 389-397.

Knook, D.L. and Sleyster, E.Ch. (1978). Lysosomes in Kupffer cells isolated from young and old rats. In *Liver and Aging* (K. Kitani, ed.) pp. 241-250, Elsevier/North-Holland Biomedical Press, Amsterdam, New York, Oxford.

Kraus, B. and Cain, H. (1974). Uber eine spontane nephropathie bei Wistar-ratten: die licht und elektronenmikroskopischen glomerulum veranderungen. *Virchow Arch. Pathol. Anat. Histol.* 363, 343.

Kroker, R., Hegner, D. and Anwer, M.S. (1980). Altered hepatobiliary transport of taurocholic acid in aged rats. *Mech. Ageing Dev.* 12, 367-373.

Lakatta, E.G. (1979). Alterations in the cardiovascular system that occur in advanced age. *Fed. Proc.* 38, 163-167.

Latini, R., Bonati, M., Marzi, E., Tacconi, M.T., Sadurska, B. and Bizzi, A. (1980). Caffeine disposition and effects in young and one-year-old rats. *J. Pharmacol.* 32, 596-599.

Massie, H.R., Colacicco, J.R. and Aiello, V.R. (1980). Phenytoin-induced serum copper and ceruloplasmin in C57BL/6J mice of different ages. *Age* 3, 33-37.

Maunderly, J.L. (1979). Effect of age on pulmonary structure and function of immature and adult animals and man. *Fed. Proc.* 38, 173-177.

McIntyre, N., Mulligan, R. and Carson, E. (1973). A critical re-evaluation. In *The Liver, Quantitative Aspects of Structure and Function*, Proceedings of First International Symposium, Swiss Society of Gastroenterology. (R. Presig and G. Paumgartener, eds.) pp. 417-426. S. Karger, Basel.

McMartin, D.N., O'Connor, J.A., Jr., Fasco, M.J. and Kaminsky, L.S. (1980). Influence of aging and induction of rat liver and kidney microsomal mixed function oxidase systems. *Toxicol. Appl. Pharmacol.* 54, 411-419.

Meihuizen, S.P. and Blansjaar, N. (1980). Stereological analysis of liver parenchymal cells from young and old rats. *Mech. Ageing Dev.* 13, 111-118.

Moloney, W.C., Boschetti, A.E. and King, V.P. (1970). Spontaneous leukemia in Fischer rats. *Cancer Res.* 30, 40-43.

Nolen, G.A. (1972). Effect of various restricted dietary regimes on the growth, health and longevity of albino rats. *J. Nutr.* 102, 1477-1493.

Pardon, I.S. and Jones, T.W.G. (1978). Barbiturate pharmacokinetics in aging tolerant mice. In *Liver and Aging* (K. Kitani, ed.) pp. 301-310, Elsevier/North-Holland Biomedical Press, Amsterdam, New York, Oxford.

Pardon, I.S., Jones, T.W.G. and Hawcroft, D.M. (1977). The apparent absence of an age-dependent lag period for hepatic enzyme induction in mice under chronic phenobarbitone treatment. In *Liver and Ageing* (D. Platt, ed.) pp. 183-193, F.K. Schattauer Verlag, Stuttgart, New York.

Paterniti, J.R., Jr., Lin, C.P. and Beattie, D.S. (1980). Regulation of heme metabolism during senescence: activity of several heme-containing enzymes and heme oxygenase in the liver and kidney of aging rats. *Mech. Ageing Dev.* 12, 80-90.

Penzes, L. (1974). Further data on the age-dependent intestinal absorption of dibasic amino acids. *Exp. Gerontol.* 9, 259-262.

Penzes, L. and Boross, M. (1974). Intestinal absorption of some heterocyclic and aromatic amino acids from the aging gut. *Exp. Gerontol.* 9, 253-258.

Peters, J.M. and Boyd, E.M.. (1967). The influence of sex and age in albino rats given a daily oral dose of caffeine at a high dose level. *Can. J. Physiol. Pharmacol.* 45, 305-311.

Pieri, C., Giuli, C., Piantanelli, L., Del Moro, M. and Fabris, N. (1978). Discussion of I. Zs. Nagy in *Liver and Aging* (K. Kitani, ed.). pp. 35-37. Elsevier/North-Holland Biomedical Press, Amsterdam, New York, Oxford.

Pieri, C., Nagy, I. Zs., Mazzufferi, G. and Giuli, C. (1975). The aging of rat liver as revealed by electron microscopic morphometry - I. Basic parameters. *Exp. Gerontol.* 10, 291-304.

Platt, D. (1977). Age dependent morphological and biochemical studies of the normal and injured rat liver. In *Liver and Ageing* (D. Platt, ed.), pp. 75-83, F.K. Schattauer Verlag, Stuttgart, New York.

Platt, D., Forster, K. and Forster, L. (1978). Age dependent kinetic studies of cytoplasmic and lysosomal enzymes of the normal and D-galactosamine injured rat liver. *Mech. Ageing Dev.* 7, 183-188.

Player, T.J., Mills, D.J. and Horton, A.A. (1977). Age-dependent changes in rat liver microsomal and mitochondrial NADPH-dependent lipid peroxidation. *Biochem. Biophys. Res. Commun.* 78, 1397-1402.

Ponomarkov, V. and Tomatis, L. (1976). The effect of long-term administration of phenobarbitone in CF-1 mice. *Cancer Lett.*, 1, 165-172.

Praaning-van Dalen, D.P., Brouwer, A. and Knook, D.L. (1981). Clearance capacity of rat liver Kupffer, endothelial, and parenchymal cells. *Gastroenterology* 81, 1036-1044.

Ribelin, W.E. and McCoy, J.R. (1965). Pathology of *Laboratory Animals*, Charles C. Thomas, Springfield.

Ricca, G.A., L, U, D.SH., Conigho, J.J., and Richardson, A.G. (1979). Rates of protein synthesis by hepatocytes isolated from rats of various ages. J. *Cell Physiol.* 97, 77-90.

Richey, D.P. and Bender, D.A. (1977). Pharmacokinetic consequences of aging. *Ann. Rev. Pharmacol. Toxicol.* 17, 49-65.

Ritzmann, R.F. and Springer, A. (1980). Age-differences in brain sensitivity and tolerance to ethanol in mice. *Age* 3, 15-17.

Roe, F.J.C. (1965). Spontaneous tumors in rats and mice. *Food Cosmet. Toxicol.* 3, 707-720.

Rolsten, C., Claghorn, J. and Samorajski, T. (1979). Long-term treatment with clozapine on aging mice. *Life Sci.* 25, 865-872.

Ross, M.H. (1961). Length of life and nutrition in the rat. *J. Nutr.* 75, 197-210.

Ross, M.H. and Bras, G. (1965). Tumor incidence patterns and nutrition in the rat. *J. Nutr.* 87, 245-260.

Ross, M.H. and Bras, G. (1973). Influence of protein under and over-nutrition on spontaneous tumor prevalence in the rat. *J. Nutr.* 103, 944-963.

Ross, M.H., Lustbader, E. and Bras, G. (1976). Dietary practices and growth responses as predictors of longevity. *Nature (London)*, 262, 548-553.

Sanadi, D.R. (1978). Metabolic changes and their significance in aging. In *The Hand book of the Biology of Aging.* (C.E. Caleb and L. Hayflick, eds.) pp. 73-98, van Nostrand Reinhold Company, New York.

Schlettwein-Gsell, D. (1970). Survival curves of an old age rat colony. *Gerontologia* 16, 111-115.

Schmucker, D.L. (1979). Age-related changes in drug disposition. *Pharmacol. Rev.* 30, 445-456.

Schmucker, D.L., Mooney, J. and Jones, A. (1977). Age-related changes in the hepatic endoplasmic reticulum: a quantitative analysis. *Science* 197, 1005-1008.

Schmucker, D.L. and Wang, R.K. (1980). Age-related changes in liver drug-metabolizing enzymes. *Exp. Gerontol.* 15, 321-329.

Sharp, J.G., Riches, A.C., Littlewood, V. and Thoma, D.B. (1976). The incidence, pathology and transplantation of hepatomas in CBA mice. *J. Pathol.* 119, 211-220.

Shima, A. and Sugahara, T. (1976). Age-dependent ploidy class changes in mouse hepatocyte nuclei as revealed by Feulgen-DNA cytofluorometry. *Exp. Gerontol.* 11, 193-203.

Shock, N.W. (1979). Systems physiology and aging. Introduction. *Fed. Proc.* 38, 161-162.

Sirica, A.E. and Pitot, H.C. (1980). Drug metabolism and effects of carcinogens in cultured hepatic cells. *Pharmacol. Rev.* 31, 205-228.

Slanina, P. and Stalhandske, T. (1977). *In vitro* metabolism of nicotine in liver of ageing mice. *Arch. Int. Pharmacodyn.* 226, 258-262.

Snell, K.C. (1967). Renal disease of the rat. In *Pathology of Laboratory Rats and Mice* (E. Cotchin and F.J.C. Roe, eds.) pp. 105-147, Blackwell Scientific Publications, Oxford and Edinburgh.

Stohs, S.J., Al-Turk, W.A. and Hassing, J.M. (1980). Altered drug metabolism in hepatic and extrahepatic tissues in mice as a function of age. *Age* 3, 88-92.

Storer, J.B. (1966). Longevity and gross pathology at death in 22 inbred mouse strains. *J. Gerontol.* 21, 404-409.

Sun, A.Y. and Samorajski, T. (1975). The effects of age and alcohol on $(Na^+ + K^+)$-ATPase activity of whole homogenate and synaptosomes prepared from mouse and human brain. *J. Neurochem.* 24, 161-164.

Thompson, S.W., Huseby, R.A., Fox, M.A., Davis, C.L. and Hunt, R.D. (1961). Spontaneous tumors in the Sprague-Dawley rat. *J. Nat. Cancer Inst.* 27, 1037-1057.

Thurman, R.G. and Kauffman, F.C. (1980). Factors regulating drug metabolism in intact hepatocytes. *Pharmacol. Rev.* 31, 229-251.

Tomatis, L., Turusov, V., Charles, R.T. and Boicchi, M. (1974). Effect of long-term exposure to 1,1-dichloro-2,2-bis(p-chlorophenyl)ethylene, to 1,1-dichloro-2,2-bis(p-chlorophenyl)ethane, and to the two chemicals combined on CF-1 mice. *J. Nat. Cancer Inst.* 52, 883-891.

Tucker, S.M., Mason, R.L. and Beauchene, R.E. (1976). Influence of diet and feed restriction on kidney function of aging male rats. *J. Gerontol.* 31, 264-270.

Turusov, V.S., ed. (1973). Pathology of tumors. In *Laboratory Animals* IARC Sci. Publ. No. 5, Vol. I, Part I. Int. Agency Res. Cancer, Lyon.

Turusov, V.S., ed. (1976). Pathology of tumors. In *Laboratory Animals* IARC Sci. Publ. No. 6, Vol. I, Part 2. Int. Agency Res. Cancer, Lyon.

van Bezooijen, C.F.A. (1978). Cellular basis of liver aging studied with isolated hepatocytes. Ph.D. Thesis, University of Utrecht, The Netherlands.

van Bezooijen, C.F.A., Grell, T. and Knook, D.L. (1976). Albumin synthesis by liver parenchymal cells isolated from young, adult and old rats. *Biochem. Biophys. Res. Commun.* 71, 513-519.

van Bezooijen, C.F.A., Grell, T. and Knook, D.L. (1977). The effect of age on protein synthesis by isolated liver parenchymal cells. *Mech. Ageing Dev.* 6, 293-304.

van Bezooijen, C.F.A. and Knook, D.L. (1978). A comparison of age-related changes in bromosulfophalein metabolism in the liver and isolated hepatocytes. In *Liver and Aging* (K. Kitani, ed.) pp. 131-141, Elsevier/North-Holland Biomedical Press, Amsterdam, New York, Oxford.

van Bezooijen, C.F.A., Sakkee, A.N. and Knook, D.L. (1981). Sex and strain dependency of age-related changes in protein synthesis of isolated rat hepatocytes. *Mech. Ageing Dev.* 17, 11-18.

van Bezooijen, C.F.A., Soekawa, Y., Ohta, M., Nokubo, M. and Kitani, K. (1980). Metabolism of digitoxin by isolated rat hepatocytes. *Biochem. Pharmacol.* 29, 3023-3025.

van Steenis, G. and Kroes, R. (1971). Changes in the nervous system and musculature of old rats. *Vet. Pathol.* 8, 320-332.

Varga, F. and Fischer, E. (1978). Age dependent changes in blood supply of the liver and in the biliary excretion of eosin in rats. In *Liver and Aging* (K. Kitani, ed.) pp. 327-339. Elsevier/North-Holland Biomedical Press, Amsterdam, New York, Oxford.

Verzar, F. (1961). The age of the individual as one of the parameters of pharmacological action. *Acta Physiol. Acad. Hungaric.* 19, 313-318.

Vesell, E.S. (1980). Why individuals vary in their response to drugs. *TIPS* 1980, 349-351.

Vestal, R.E. (1978). Drug use in the elderly: A review of problems and special con siderations. *Drugs* 16, 358-382.

Viskup, R.W., Baker, M., Hobrook, J.P. and Penniall, R. (1979). Age-associated changes in activities of rat hepatocytes, I. Protein synthesis. *Exp. Aging Res.* 5, 487-495.

von Wittenau, M.S. and Gans, D.J. (1981). Aging as a confounding factor in car cinogenicity bioassays. *Drug Chem. Toxicol.* 4, 307-310.

Wang, R.K.J. and Mays, L.L. (1977). Opposite changes in rat liver glucose-6-phosphate dehydrogenase during aging in Sprague-Dawley and Fischer 344 male rats. *Exp. Gerontol.* 12, 117-124.

Ward, J.M. and Vlahakis, G. (1978). Evaluation of hepatocellular neoplasms in mice. *J. Nat. Cancer Inst.* 61, 807-811.

Webb, J. and Bailey, E. (1975). Changes in activities of some enzymes associated with hepatic lipogenesis in the rat from weaning to old age and the effect of sucrose feeding. *Int. J. Biochem.* 6, 813.

Wheeler, H.0., Meltzer, J.I. and Bradley, S.E. (1969). Biliary transport and hepatic storage of sulfobromophthalein sodium in the unanesthetized dog, in normal man, and in patients with hepatic disease. *J. Clin. Invest.* 39, 1131-1143.

Wiberg, G.S., Trenholm, H.L. and Coldwell, B.B. (1970). Increased ethanol toxicity in old rats: changes in LD_{50}, *in vivo* and *in vitro* metabolism, and liver alchohol dehydrogenase activity. *Toxicol. Appl. Pharmacol.* 16, 718-727.

Wilson, P.D. (1972). Enzyme changes in ageing mammals. *Gerontologia* 18, 36-54.

Index